Fifty Years of Findings from the Jefferson Longitudinal Study of Medical Education

Joseph S. Gonnella • Clara A. Callahan
J. Jon Veloski • Jennifer DeSantis
Mohammadreza Hojat

Fifty Years of Findings from the Jefferson Longitudinal Study of Medical Education

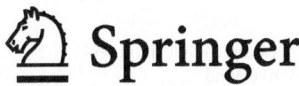 Springer

Joseph S. Gonnella
Sidney Kimmel Medical College
Thomas Jefferson University
Philadelphia, PA, USA

Clara A. Callahan
Sidney Kimmel Medical College
Thomas Jefferson University
Philadelphia, PA, USA

J. Jon Veloski
Sidney Kimmel Medical College
Thomas Jefferson University
Philadelphia, PA, USA

Jennifer DeSantis
Sidney Kimmel Medical College
Thomas Jefferson University
Philadelphia, PA, USA

Mohammadreza Hojat
Sidney Kimmel Medical College
Thomas Jefferson University
Philadelphia, PA, USA

ISBN 978-3-030-85381-5   ISBN 978-3-030-85379-2   (eBook)
https://doi.org/10.1007/978-3-030-85379-2

This Springer imprint is published by the registered company Springer Nature Switzerland AG
The registered company address is: Gewerbestrasse 11, 6330 Cham, Switzerland

Foreword

What you have in your hand (or on your desktop) is a remarkable document. For 50 years, Jefferson has conducted a series of studies of virtually every aspect of the process and outcome of medical education. It provides far more than a snapshot of the going-on in a medical school; it is more like an IMAX theatre presentation of the journey from applicant to student to resident to physician. A total of 204 publications have resulted, spanning all aspects of medical education.

I am honored to have been asked to write this foreword. As it happens, the duration of the program almost precisely spans the duration of my professional career. It began in the late 1960s and early 1970s; I started in medical education in 1971. We have observed and participated in the progress in medical education together for the past five decades. But I have to confess some ignorance of the JLS. Before I read the book, I was dimly aware of the existence of the program, as I imagine most people in the field are. I knew some of the key players, Joe Gonnella, Jon Veloski, and Mohammadreza Hojat, and have seen them present on numerous occasions. I was honored to visit Jefferson as a guest of Joe Gonnella many years ago. But until I saw the totality of studies laid out for me when I took on this assignment, I really had no idea how comprehensive the JLS was.

I have been searching for a metaphor. Calling it a "bible" of medical education is, frankly, hackneyed and imprecise. The bible is grouped by author, and there is no grand design (at least as furnished by mortals). I think a more appropriate metaphor is a Chinese restaurant menu, probably the most extensive menu you have ever come across. It contains just about every part of animal or vegetable. Many are familiar (honey garlic spareribs) and many others are not (duck palms). There are natural groupings by meal component—appetizer and dessert—and source—chicken, duck, etc. And there are hundreds of options. Some you might have thought of and many you have not.

So it is for the abstracts in this book. There are natural groupings—admissions, clinical evaluations, and specialization—and there are studies that could likely be anticipated—old vs. new MCAT and predictive validity of clerkship ratings. But there are other studies that are both novel and critical, such as the decline in empathy in medical school (See Chapter 5) and the relation between disciplinary action by boards and performance in medical school (Chapter 7).

A central element of the study is the longitudinal database, and many studies, such as predictive validity of MCAT or studies of clinical performance ratings (Chapter 3), come naturally out of a longitudinal database collected on medical students. But many studies go beyond the data contained in the database (Chapter 4), and which examines predictors of rural practice, or research which looks at global ratings and ACGME competencies (Chapter 3), or the studies of psychosocial attributes (Chapter 5), career expectations (Chapter 4), and personality (Chapters 4 and 5). Indeed, an outstanding example of studies that extend beyond the database are the studies using the Jefferson Scale of Empathy and that have, in turn, spawned hundreds of studies at many other institutions (see Preface).

I think this is a critical aspect of the longitudinal study. Far too frequently, longitudinal studies are defined and circumscribed by the database designed at the inception of the study. If a variable is not in the database, it is not studied. But, in my experience, this is putting the cart before the horse. It is simply not possible to envision from the outset what variables may be needed to address specific questions. As a consequence, most databases have many variables that never see the light of day, yet the critical variables you need to address a specific question are not there.

A review of the studies in this book clearly shows a far more comprehensive and hypothesis-driven strategy. Studies arise to address specific questions. They may be answered directly from the existing data (MCAT and medical school performance, Chapter 1) or may require additional data capture (empathy and admission essays, Chapter 6). This is a critically important message in these days of "big data." While it is hard to design a database, get buy-in from all the actors, input all the data, clean it, and debug it; that is only part of the job. If you constrain your research to questions that can be answered from the data that is "in there," the utility of the database will be limited. Rather, the design must have the flexibility to incorporate additional measures arising from ongoing studies. And the process of generating hypotheses and designing studies cannot be limited to what you already have in hand.

What will the reader get from this book? Well, to begin with, a profound sense of awe at the quality and quantity of research that the JLS has produced. Second, a detailed study of each abstract should provide many examples of unique and creative approaches to study questions, research designs, and analyses. Finally, but perhaps most importantly, is an understanding of the factors that enabled this unique research program that, on the one hand, remains focused on the institution, based on the premise that "medical schools have a social responsibility and ethical obligation to monitor the quality of their educational programs, to assess their educational outcomes, and to ensure that their educational goals have been achieved for the purposes of public safety," but on the other makes a substantial contribution to the medical education research community at large.

Geoffrey Norman,
McMaster University
Hamilton, ON, Canada

Preface

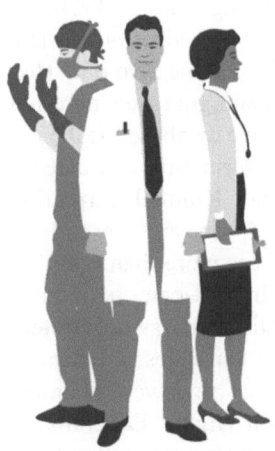

The Jefferson Longitudinal Study of Medical Education: 50 Years of Research and Service

The Jefferson Longitudinal Study of Medical Education (JLSMED) came into existence 50 years ago. To date, it is the most comprehensive, extensive, and uninterrupted longitudinal study of medical students and graduates maintained in a single medical school. The study was based on the conviction that medical schools have a social responsibility and ethical obligation to monitor the quality of their educational programs, to assess their educational outcomes, and to ensure that their educational goals have been achieved for the purposes of public safety. The title of "longitudinal study" was chosen because of the intention to follow all medical students from the time of matriculation to the time of graduation, through graduate medical training, and throughout their entire active professional careers to monitor the short- and long-term effects of medical education.

A Historical Perspective

The original home of the JLSMED was the *Office of Medical Education*, later renamed the *Center for Research in Medical Education and Health Care*. In 2019, it became the *Asano-Gonnella Center for Research in Medical Education and Health Care* in recognition of the generosity of Dr. Yoshihisa Asano, the founder and chairman emeritus of the Noguchi Medical Research Institute, Tokyo, Japan, in supporting our research in the humanities and the art of medicine, and in appreciation of Joseph S. Gonnella, M.D., the founder of the Center, for his leadership role in medical education research.

Although the JLSMED was initiated in 1970, pertinent data were collected retrospectively throughout the early 1970s for students who had entered Jefferson Medical College beginning in 1964. The database expanded, beginning with the entering class of 1966 (graduating class of 1970), to include measures of clinical competence at Jefferson and after graduation at the end of the first residency year. During the early phases, both retrospective data (for graduates prior to 1970) and prospective data (for students and graduates enrolled in 1970 and thereafter) were maintained in one comprehensive database. At the present time (January 2021), this database contains academic information and career outcomes for 13,343 medical students and graduates of Sidney Kimmel (formerly Jefferson) Medical College of Thomas Jefferson University. There are presently 502 variables in the JLSMED analytic database that encompass more than 6 million data points. Data security is guided by policies developed in the Center to maintain strict confidentiality of individual data. The JLSMED data are password protected and only a few authorized professional staff of the Center can access the database.

The Accreditation Team that reviewed Thomas Jefferson University for the Middle States Commission on Higher Education praised the University for the JLSMED and made the following comment that the Center and the College are "*…to be commended for their academic interest in outcome data, responsiveness to faculty and department needs, and the clear use of data to modify the curriculum and teaching environment …The Center continues to track data from a large number of sources before, during, and after students' tenure at the College. Their use of this data has impacted many components of the curriculum, the learning environment, individual student development, and program planning ….*"

Goals of the Jefferson Longitudinal Study

The general goals of the JLSMED can be described in two words: *service* and *research*. Service is rendered to the college's administration, faculty, and academic committees by providing them with information to assist their decision-making regarding academic programs. Service is also provided to students by identifying those who may need remedial assistance to perform at their fullest potential.

Information from the database is also used in conducting research. Specific goals of the JLSMED are described as follows:

1. To provide data to the College's administration, for example by preparing statistics for the Center's annual report; retrieving information on an individual student's performance compared to class performance for inclusion in the Dean's Medical School Performance Evaluation; assessing the College's educational programs and policies; preparing self-evaluation information as requested by the Liaison Committee on Medical Education for accreditation; and responding to inquiries by faculty and senior administrators

2. To provide objective information to the College's academic committees (e.g., Admissions, Student Promotion, and Curriculum) and to respond in a timely manner to the faculty members' inquiries related to their institutional and academic interests

3. To provide up-to-date information to the Office of Student Affairs and Career Counseling and to prepare predictions about students who may need supplementary education, in order to better prepare them for licensure examinations and the challenges of medical school

4. To address empirically and systematically a variety of complex and contemporary issues raised by researchers

5. To disseminate research findings through presentations at national and international professional meetings and publications in peer-reviewed journals for a broader audience

The Scope of the Jefferson Longitudinal Study Database

The information encoded in the database is routinely updated. Variables have been added or archived in response to changes in curriculum. Despite this dynamic nature, some central constructs (e.g., performance measures prior to, during, and beyond medical school) and their corresponding variables have remained relatively unaltered. Examples of such variables are performance scores on the nationally administered standardized tests or examinations taken before medical school (e.g., the Scholastic Aptitude Test [SAT], the Medical College Admission Test [MCAT]), during medical school (e.g., assessments of acquisition of clinical knowledge and rating of clinical competence in third-year core clerkships, performance on medical licensing examinations), and after medical school (e.g., specialty choice, licensing, and board certification status).

Some medical schools have expressed interest in learning more about the JLSMED, requesting copies of the questionnaires used in the study and information about how to set up a longitudinal study and needed resources. In response to a request from *Academic Medicine* in 2011, we prepared and published in that journal a schematic snapshot of the JLSMED for those interested in a model for the development of a longitudinal study of medical students and graduates (Appendix A).

An important feature of the JLSMED is the collection of clinical competence ratings of graduates made by the program director at the end of the first year of residency training. This point in time, the end of the first postgraduate training year, was deliberately chosen to capture the impact of medical school education while minimizing the inevitable effect of the residency experience on competence ratings. Furthermore, at this point, the directors of residency programs would have had sufficient opportunities to observe a resident's professional behavior in a variety of clinical situations to make an informed judgment. The Postgraduate Competence Rating Form was developed to assess graduates' competence in the science and the art of medicine and demonstration of the three roles of physicians, as a *clinician, teacher, and manager of resources* (a copy of the Postgraduate Competence Rating Form is shown in Appendix B).

All the variables in the JLSMED database can be grouped into three categories:

1. *Data before education at Jefferson,* which include demographic, academic, and other admission data.
2. *Data during education at Jefferson,* which include course grades; ratings of clinical competence in the third-year clerkships; hospitals of clerkships; performance on Steps 1 and 2 of the United States Medical Licensing Examination (USMLE, formerly the National Board of Medical Examiners' examinations); coded reasons for any change in academic status (transfer, dismissal, delayed graduation); and responses to the entrance and exit questionnaires on attitudes, personal qualities, future plans, and preferences.
3. *Data after graduation from Jefferson,* which include geographic location and hospitals of residency, specialties pursued in residency training, ratings of postgraduate clinical competence, performance on Step 3 of the USMLE (formerly Part III of the National Board of Medical Examiners' examination), geographic location and specialty after residency, board certification status, types of professional activities, faculty appointments, changes of practice and location, etc. In addition, follow-up questionnaires have solicited graduates' evaluation of their education at Jefferson, their professional concerns, perceived problems, types of activities, types of patients, and research productivities. The scope of the JLSMED database is depicted in Appendix A.

Current Faculty and Staff of the Center Involved in the Jefferson Longitudinal Study

- **Joseph S. Gonnella, M.D.**, Founder, Dean Emeritus, and Distinguished Professor of Medicine
- **Clara A. Callahan, M.D.**, Emeritus Director of the Center, and the Lillian H. Brent Dean of Student and Admission, and Professor of Pediatrics

- **Vittorio Maio, Pharm.D.**, Managing Director of the Center, Research Professor, Jefferson College of Population Health, Director, Health Economics and Outcomes Research Fellowship, Jefferson College of Population Health
- **J. Jon Veloski, M.S.**, Director of Medical Education Research, Instructor, Department of Psychiatry and Human Behavior
- **Mohammadreza Hojat, Ph.D.**, Director of the Jefferson Longitudinal Study, Research Professor, Department of Psychiatry and Human Behavior
- **Aaron Douglas, Ph.D.**, Associate Director of the Jefferson Longitudinal Study
- **Jennifer DeSantis, M.Ed.**, Senior Research Study Analyst
- **Lifan He, M.S.**, Programmer/Analyst
- **Phyllis M. Accetta**, Administrative Assistant
- **Shira Carroll**, Administrative Assistant
- **Edward Nicks, Jr.**, Statistical Data Coordinator

The JLSMED could not have survived without the willingness and participation of those who cooperated and shared information with us. First and foremost, we gratefully appreciate the cooperation of thousands of our students and graduates who have participated in the study by completing our surveys and granting us permission to collect clinical competence ratings on their behalf from their postgraduate program directors. The offices of Admissions, Registrar, and Alumni have always been helpful in providing us with data. Professional organizations such as the Association of American Medical Colleges (AAMC) and the American Medical Association (AMA) have routinely and continuously provided us with information about our graduates. Finally, we would like to express our sincere gratitude to the directors of residency training programs in more than 700 hospitals and residency training institutions all over the USA who have completed our postgraduate rating form on behalf of our graduates.

Grouping the Jefferson Longitudinal Study Publications in Different Chapters

The JLSMED has been used to address a variety of issues in medical education. Because of this variety, the grouping of the studies into homogeneous chapters was not an easy task. After considering several options, we decided to classify the published studies into the following seven chapters:

1. *Admissions* (e.g., standardized tests, academic preparation, and other admission variables)
2. *Demographics* (e.g., gender, age, race)
3. *Medical School Evaluations* (preclinical and clinical)
4. *Postgraduate and Career* (e.g., clinical competence, specialization, professional activities)

5. *Psychosocial Attributes* (e.g., personal qualities, personality measures, indicators of well-being, and early life experiences)
6. *Professionalism* (e.g., measuring empathic orientation in patient care, interprofessional collaboration, and lifelong learning)
7. Miscellaneous (publications that could not be grouped into the aforementioned categories, such as interviews, letters to the editors, commentaries, and editorials)

Some of the studies could have been included in more than one chapter (e.g., gender difference on academic performance or psychosocial attributes). Despite this overlap, the abstract of each study in this book appears in only one chapter, based on the main focus of the study. Abstracts of the studies that have been published in professional journals are presented in alphabetical order by the authors' names in each subsection. Overall, there were a total of 204 publications relevant to the JLSMED. The book authors were listed as coauthors of 194 of these publications. The majority of these abstract entries reported ($n = 167$) are indeed reprints of the published articles in peer-reviewed journals. We obtained permission from journal publishers through Copyright Clearance Center to reprint the abstracts. We would like to thank the Copyright Clearance Center for providing us with the facility to contact journal publishers and also publishers that kindly granted us permission to reprint the published abstracts. Some journal publishers required that the link to the article be printed and/or copyright acknowledgment appear along with the abstract. We had difficulties in obtaining permission or in contacting publishers of five articles; abstracts of these articles were rewritten by us. Some publications did not have abstracts in their original publication (e.g., interviews, letters to the editor, editorials, commentaries ($n = 28$)). We drafted brief abstracts for such publications for the book.

Productivity of the Jefferson Longitudinal Study

The JLSMED is the most prolific longitudinal study of medical students and graduates of a single medical school. This longitudinal study has resulted in 204 publications (as of January 2021) in peer-reviewed journals, listed in the bibliography section at the end of this book. Some of those studies were also presented before national or international professional meetings prior to their publication. We (JSG, JJV, MH, and James B. Erdmann, Ph.D.) served as the invited editors for a thematic issue of *Academic Medicine* on "*Assessment Measures in Medical School, Residency, and Beyond: The Connections*" (*Academic Medicine*, Supplement No. 2, Volume 68, February 1993). This supplement subsequently was published as an independent book by Springer Publishing Company. Also, in 1999, we (JSG, JJV, MH, and Gang Xu) were invited to serve as the guest editors of a special section of *Evaluation & the Health Professions* on the topic of "*Medical Education and the Changes in Health Care*" (Volume 22, No. 2, June 1999). We (JJV, MH) were also invited to write a chapter on the measurement of professionalism in medicine in a book edited by Dr. David Stern of the University of Michigan, in which we describe three scales, developed as offshoots of the JLSMED (*Jefferson Scale of Empathy, Jefferson Scale of Physician-Nurse Collaboration,* and *Jefferson Scale of Physician Lifelong Learning*) to be operational measures of core elements of professionalism in medicine (Veloski & Hojat, 2006).

Information about the JLSMED is routinely updated and posted on the website of the Asano-Gonnella Center for Research in Medical Education and Health Care.

- Click on the following link for updated general information about the Asano-Gonnella Center for Research in Medical Education and Health Care: http://www.jefferson.edu/university/skmc/research/research-medical-education.html. Jefferson.edu/CRMEHC
- Click on the following link for updated information on the Jefferson Longitudinal Study: https://www.jefferson.edu/academics/colleges-schools-institutes/skmc/research/research-medical-education/longitudinal-study-medical-education.html
- Click on the following link for updated information about the Jefferson Scale of Empathy and related research findings: https://www.jefferson.edu/academics/colleges-schools-institutes/skmc/research/research-medical-education/jefferson-scale-of-empathy.html

We have developed the following ten psychometrically sound instruments as by-products of the JLSMED for the assessment of medical education outcomes, professional development of physicians in training and in practice, and patient outcomes. We have reported convincing evidence to support the psychometrics (e.g., validity and reliability) of these instruments:

1. **Jefferson Scale of Empathy (JSE-S** version for administration to medical students, 20 items)
2. **Jefferson Scale of Empathy (JSE-HPS** version for administration to all health professions students other than medicine, 20 items)
3. **Jefferson Scale of Empathy (JSE-HP** version, for administration to all practicing health professionals, 20 items)
4. **Jefferson Scale of Patient Perception of Physician Empathy (JSPPPE,** for administration to patients, 5 items)
5. **Jefferson Scale of Attitudes Toward Physician-Nurse Collaboration** (15 items)
6. **Scale of Attitudes Toward Physician-Pharmacist Collaboration** (16 items)
7. **Jefferson Scale of Attitudes Toward Interprofessional Collaboration (JeffSATIC,** 20 items)
8. **Jefferson Scale of Physician Lifelong Learning (JeffSPLL,** for administration to physicians, 14 items)
9. **Jefferson Scale of Physician Lifelong Learning (JeffSPLL-MS** version for administration to medical students, 14 items)
10. **Scale of Overall Satisfaction with Primary Care Physicians** (10 items)

These instruments have already attracted the attention of many researchers from the USA and abroad, evidenced by the increasing number of requests we have been receiving for permission to use them. For example, as of January 2021, we have received over 2200 requests by researchers from 89 countries for permission to use the Jefferson Scale of Empathy. This scale has already been translated into 56 languages, and we have a list of 424 publications from national and international researchers outside of Jefferson (as of January 2021) in the English language in peer-reviewed journals in which the Jefferson Scale of Empathy has been used or reviewed, and the list is growing. This list is posted on the following link: https://www.jefferson.edu/content/dam/academic/skmc/crmehc/8.27.21_Bibliography_Natl-Intl%20researchers.pdf.

Final Remarks

In summary, medical schools should be responsible for collecting pertinent data with which to monitor their educational programs and to assess their educational outcomes for public safety and advancement of the science and art of medicine. We hope that this book can help medical schools to recognize the value of longitudinal research as a means to discharge the aforementioned responsibilities. The quality of the medical education and the cost should always be monitored. Our recent 50th anniversary review of the Penn State-Jefferson accelerated combined BS-MD degree program (Gonnella et al., 2021) indicates that it is possible to reduce the length of the journey to obtain an MD degree and thereby the cost without compromising the quality of medical education outcomes. To honor the principle of social accountability, assessments of medical education outcomes should be seen as a core mandate that must be acted upon.

Joseph S. Gonnella
Clara A. Callahan
J. Jon Veloski
Jennifer DeSantis
Mohammadreza Hojat
Philadelphia, PA, USA

References

Gonnella, J. S., Callahan, C. A., Erdmann, J. B., Veloski, J. J., Jafari, N., Markle, R. A., & Hojat, M. (2021). Preparing for the MD: How long, at what cost, and with what outcomes? *Academic Medicine, 96*(1), 101–107. https://doi.org/10.1097/ACM0000000000003298.
Veloski, J., & Hojat, M. (2006). Measuring specific elements of professionalism: Empathy, teamwork, and lifelong learning. In D.T. Stern (Ed.). *Measuring medical professionalism.* (pp. 117–145). Oxford: Oxford University Press.

Appendix A

AM Last Page: The Jefferson Longitudinal Study of Medical Education

Joseph S. Gonnella, MD, founder and director, Center for Research in Medical Education and Health Care; Mohammadreza Hojat, PhD, director, Jefferson Longitudinal Study; Jon Veloski, MS, director, Medical Education Division, Center for Research in Medical Education and Health Care, Jefferson Medical College of Thomas Jefferson University

Data Available by Matriculating Class

	1964	1970	1980	1990	2000	2010
Demographic and academic*						
Clinical clerkship		1972				
Residency	1966					
Career outcomes						
Psychosocial				1992		
Jefferson Scale of Empathy					2002	

*Demographic and academic data for the classes of 1964-1969 were extr-acted retrospectively.

Scope of Database

Before Medical School
- Demographics
- SAT scores
- GPA science
- GPA nonscience
- MCAT scores

During Medical School
- Matriculation surveys ⎤ 1st Year
- Course grades
- GPA
- Course grades ⎤ 2nd Year
- GPA
- NBE/USMLE 1
- Examination grades ⎤ 3rd Year
- Clerkship ratings
- Hospitals of clerkships
- GPA
- NBE/USMLE 2 ⎤ 4th Year
- Graduation survey
- Permission form

After Medical School
- Residency specialty ⎤ PGY-
- Residency institution
- Geographic location
- Rating of competency
- NBE/USMLE 3

- Specialty ⎤ Career
- Geographic location
- Board certification
- Faculty appointment
- Type of practice
- Active status
- Follow-up surveys

Reason for initiating the study: The Jefferson Longitudinal Study (JLS) at Jefferson Medical College of Thomas Jefferson University was initiated in 1970 based on the premise that medical schools have an obligation to society to monitor their educational outcomes. [1,2]

History: The JLS was implemented with an intention to track every Jefferson medical student throughout his or her entire professional career. Data for the JLS are routinely updated for all entering classes from 1964 to the present using information from the Association of American Medical Colleges, American Medical Association, American Board of Medical Specialties, National Board of Medical Examiners, and in-house sources. The JLS retrieves information from the most comprehensive, extensive, and uninterrupted longitudinal database of medical students and graduates maintained in a single medical school.

Goals

Service to
- Faculty (e.g., responding to inquiries)
- Academic committees (e.g., providing data to analyze admissions trends, to evaluate programs, or to examine success/failure factors in students' performance)
- College/dean's office/administrators (e.g., providing data for the annual report, dean's letters of evaluations, or accreditation)
- Students (e.g., guiding academic and career development)

Research
- Data analyses in collaboration with faculty to support their scholarship and address issues in medical education for publication and presentation at professional meetings

By the Numbers

As of December 2010, the JLS
- Contained approximately 6 million pieces of data
- Tracked 10,600 students
- Garnered data from 573 postgraduate training hospitals
- Inspired 179 peer-reviewed publications* (56 in *Academic Medicine*)

* Abstracts of 155 publications of the JLS are posted at http://jdc.jefferson.edu/jlsme.

New Instruments

The JLS has led to the development of the following instruments for measuring educational outcomes:
- Jefferson Scale of Empathy [3]
- Jefferson Scale of Attitudes Toward Physician–Nurse Collaboration [4]
- Jefferson Scale of Physician Lifelong Learning [5]
- Scale of Attitudes Toward Physician–Pharmacist Collaboration [6]

References
1. Hojat M, Gonnella JS, Veloski JJ, Erdmann JB. Jefferson Medical College Longitudinal Study: A prototype for evaluation of changes. Educ Health. 1996;9:99-113.
2. Gonnella JS, Hojat M, Erdman JB, Veloski JJ, eds. Assessment Measures in Medical School, Residency, and Practice: The Connections. New York, NY: Springer; 1993.
3. Hojat M. Empathy in Patient Care: Antecedents, Development, Measurement, and Outcomes. New York, NY: Springer; 2007
4. Hojat M, Gonnella JS, Nasca TJ, et al. Comparisons of American, Israeli, Italian, and Mexican physicians and nurses on the total and factor scores of four dimensions of the Jefferson Scale of Attitudes Toward Physician–Nurse Collaboration. Int J Nurs Stud. 2003;40:426–435.
5. Hojat M, Veloski JJ, Gonnella JS. Measurement and correlates of physicians' lifelong learning. Acad Med. 2009;84:1066–1074. Available at: http://journals.lww.com/academicmedicine/Fulltext/2009/08000/Measurement_and_Correlates_of_Physicians_Lifelong.21.aspx. Accessed November 9, 2010.
6. Hojat M, Gonnella JS. An instrument for measuring pharmacist and physician attitudes towards collaboration: Preliminary psychometric data. J Interprof Care. 2011;25:66-72.

Appendix B

POSTGRADUATE RATING FORM

I. Please rate the resident in each of the following items by circling the appropriate number. In making the ratings please compare this resident with all residents you have supervised, not just with those in your recent group.

	Top Quarter	Upper Middle Quarter	Lower Middle Quarter	Bottom Quarter	Insufficient Information to Judge
1. Attention to collection of data related to health risks	4	3	2	1	X
2. Collection of history of the present illness from the patient or family	4	3	2	1	X
3. Ability to communicate effectively with patients and their families	4	3	2	1	X
4. Ability to act effectively in an emergency	4	3	2	1	X
5. Competence in performing physical examination	4	3	2	1	X
6. Willingness to ask for help when needed	4	3	2	1	X
7. Attention to psychological and emotional factors related to the patient's health	4	3	2	1	X
8. Use of literature in diagnosis and treatment	4	3	2	1	X
9. Documentation of reasons for obtaining laboratory data	4	3	2	1	X
10. Counseling patients about preventive care and wellness	4	3	2	1	X
11. Thoroughness of differential diagnosis	4	3	2	1	X
12. Awareness of socio-psychological factors affecting patient's condition	4	3	2	1	X
13. Ability to handle anxiety-producing situations	4	3	2	1	X
14. Adherence to professional ethical standards	4	3	2	1	X
15. Knowledge of basic science areas most closely related to postgraduate program	4	3	2	1	X
16. Judgment in implementing care	4	3	2	1	X
17. Effectiveness as a teacher of medical students and/or other health professionals	4	3	2	1	X
18. Willingness to admit an error in judgment	4	3	2	1	X
19. Willingness to proceed independently when appropriate	4	3	2	1	X
20. Relationships with other health care personnel	4	3	2	1	X
21. Thoroughness in collection of pertinent past history of the patient	4	3	2	1	X
22. Thoroughness and organization of medical records	4	3	2	1	X
23. Collection of the patient's family history	4	3	2	1	X
24. Thoroughness in obtaining information from patients or families related to the patient's chief complaint	4	3	2	1	X

II. Please rate the resident's <u>**overall**</u> performance in the following areas:

	Top Quarter	Upper Middle Quarter	Lower Middle Quarter	Bottom Quarter	Insufficient Information to Judge
1. Knowledge	4	3	2	1	X
2. Data-Gathering Skills	4	3	2	1	X
3. Clinical Judgment	4	3	2	1	X
4. Professional Attitudes	4	3	2	1	X

III. If one assumes that a physician serves not only as a clinician, but also as a patient educator and a manager of health care resources, how would you rate this resident in these areas:

	Top Quarter	Upper Middle Quarter	Lower Middle Quarter	Bottom Quarter	Insufficient Information to Judge
1. Clinician	4	3	2	1	X
2. Patient educator	4	3	2	1	X
3. Manager of health care resources	4	3	2	1	X

Please see other side~

IV. How do you rate this resident's **empathetic behavior** *(defined as an understanding of the patients' inner experiences and perspective, and a capability to communicate this understanding)* on the following 10-point scale:

Not empathetic at all   Very empathetic all the time

1 . . . . 2 . . . . 3 . . . . 4 . . . . 5 . . . . 6 . . . . 7 . . . . 8 . . . . 9 10

V. Does your hospital offer a program in this resident's specialty?

○ Yes–**If Yes**, was this resident offered further postgraduate training at your hospital?   ○ Yes   ○ No.

○ No–**If No**, if your hospital had a program in this specialty, would he or she have been offered a place at your institution?   ○ Yes   ○ No.

○ Other, please comment _____

VI. Was the resident's performance consistent with the hospital's expectation at the time of acceptance?

○ Yes, *(describe)* _____

○ No, *(describe)* _____

VII. Was the dean's letter of recommendation predictive of the resident's performance?

○ Yes, *(describe)* _____

○ No, *(describe)* _____

VIII. Does this resident have qualities you would like to see in your own physician?

○ Yes, *(describe)* _____

○ No, *(describe)* _____

Thank you again for your help with this IRB approved evaluation.
If you have any questions concerning this form, or suggestions for improvement, please contact:

Mohammadreza Hojat, PhD - (215) 955-9459

(Mohammadreza.Hojat@jefferson.edu)

Please return this form to:
Asano-Gonnella Center for Research in Medical Education and Health Care

SIDNEY KIMMEL MEDICAL COLLEGE at
THOMAS JEFFERSON UNIVERSITY
1015 Walnut Street, Suite 319
Philadelphia, PA 19107

Experts' Remarks About the Book

The Jefferson Longitudinal Study of Medical Education is a tour de force in support of the effort to understand not only what is the basis for educating physicians to deliver good medical care but moreover what are the critical factors that contribute to whether such clinicians will also be *caring* to their patients as well. From preclinical to postgraduate and beyond, this book provides a high-level view of the remarkable accomplishments over 50 years of study and the important results from this program dedicated to study the quality and outcomes of medical education from ethical and psychosocial dimensions. For medical educators and those interested in the role of empathy in health care, this book is a valued resource.

Leonard H. Calabrese
Cleveland Clinic Lerner College of Medicine
of Case Western Reserve University

Theodore F. Classen, DO
Chair of Oseopathic Research and Education
and Vice Chair, Department of Rheumatic
and Immunologic Diseases, Cleveland Clinic

A wonderful compilation of outstanding work from a superb team of scientists, this book offers critical insights throughout the continuum of medical education and across key areas of great interest. Although the project is a longitudinal study, the Jefferson medical education team has succeeded in implementing a virtuous cycle, in its truest sense, acknowledging a medical school's ethical obligation to monitor quality and assess outcomes, firmly anchoring findings with strong evidence, establishing connections to clinical competence, and feeding results back to decision makers. The team sets a high bar while providing insight and inspiration for future generations of investigators. Happy 50th!

Steven L. Kanter
President and CEO, Association of Academic
Health Centers/International, Washington, DC
Editor Emeritus of *Academic Medicine*

What you have in your hand (or on your desktop) is a remarkable document. For 50 years, Jefferson has conducted a series of studies of virtually every aspect of the process and outcome of medical education. It provides far more than a snapshot of the going-on in a medical school; it is more like an IMAX theatre presentation of the journey from applicant to student to resident to physician.

Geoffrey Norman
McMaster University
Founding Editor-in-Chief,
Advances in Health Sciences Education

A Brief Description of the Book's Cover Design and Its Artist

The cover was created by the artist Michael Natter who completed his Doctor of Medicine degree at Jefferson in 2017 and went on to a residency in internal medicine and fellowship in endocrinology at NYU Langone Health in New York City.

The figure clutching a textbook depicts a healthcare clinician at any stage of training or career. The artist chose hands as the focal point to convey empathy, thoughtfulness, and humanism. The physician's hands are needed to palpate, examine, and perform procedures, but they are also used to greet, console, and heal. Thus, the image reminds us of the nature and role of the physician.

The anatomy textbook underscores the importance of the basic medical sciences in the clinical arena. The young physician depicted never forgets this foundation of clinical competence. The timepiece is a metaphor for the Longitudinal Study. Such a time-series research design enables investigation of questions that are difficult or impossible to probe in cross-sectional studies.

Acknowledgments

We would like to thank Dr. Yoshihisa Asano, founder and president emeritus of the Noguchi Medical Research Institute, Tokyo, Japan, for his Medical Humanities Fund to Asano-Gonnella Center for Research in Medical Education and Health Care.

We would like to thank Shira Carroll for her contribution to the design, copy editing, and stylistic aspects of this book; Pamela Walter for her editorial polishing; and Timothy Flanagan for his contributions to the design of the book. We would also like to thank Lilith Dorko, senior acquisition editor of psychology and cognitive science at Springer, for her initial positive feedback to endorse the value of our book proposal and encouraging us to pursue the idea of assembling such a document from findings of the Jefferson Longitudinal Study of Medical Education.

We also thank the journal publishers that granted us permission to reprint the abstracts of the articles: The American Medical Association, American Psychiatric Publishing, Elsevier, S. Karger AG, the Massachusetts Medical Society, Sage Publications Inc., Society of Teachers of Family Medicine, Springer Nature, Taylor and Francis Group, John Wiley & Sons, Inc., and Wolters Kluwer Health, Inc.

Contents

1   Admissions 1
  1.1 Standardized Tests 4
      1.1.1 The Predictive Validity of Three Versions of the MCAT
             in Relation to Performance in Medical School,
             Residency, and Licensing Examinations: A Longitudinal
             Study of 36 Classes of Jefferson Medical College 4
      1.1.2 Science, Verbal, or Quantitative Skills: Which Is the Most
             Important Predictor of Physician Competence? 5
      1.1.3 A Validity Study of the Writing Sample Section
             of the Medical College Admission Test 6
      1.1.4 Predictive Validity of the MCAT for Students
             with Two Sets of Scores 7
      1.1.5 Delays in Completing Medical School: Predictors
             and Outcomes 8
      1.1.6 The Overall Validity of the New MCAT 9
      1.1.7 Long-Range Predictive and Differential Validities
             of the Scholastic Aptitude Test in Medical School 10
      1.1.8 Predictive Validity of the MCAT as a Function
             of Undergraduate Institutions 11
      1.1.9 The Relationship Between MCAT Science Subtest Scores
             and Performance in Medical School: The Impact
             of the Undergraduate Institution 12
  1.2 Academic Preparation 13
      1.2.1 Reexamination of Relationships Between Students'
             Undergraduate Majors, Medical School Performances,
             and Career Plans at Jefferson Medical College 13
      1.2.2 The Jefferson-Penn State BS-MD Program: A 26-Year
             Experience 14

1.2.3   Evaluation of an Enrichment Program for Entering
        Medical Students Predicted to Be in Need of Academic
        Preparation.....................................   15
1.2.4   Preparing for the MD: How Long, at What Cost,
        and with What Outcomes?.........................   16
1.2.5   Premedical Training, Personal Characteristics,
        and Performance in Medical School   17
1.2.6   Assessments of Empathy in Medical School Admissions:
        What Additional Evidence Is Needed?   18
1.2.7   Postbaccalaureate Preparation and Performance
        in Medical School   19
1.2.8   A Program to Recruit and Educate Medical Students
        to Practice Family Medicine in Underserved Areas.......   20
1.2.9   Evaluation of a Selective Medical School Admission
        Policy to Increase the Number of Family Physicians
        in Rural and Underserved Areas   21
1.2.10 Demographic, Educational, and Economic Factors
        Related to Recruitment and Retention of Physicians
        in Rural Pennsylvania   22
1.2.11 Using Postgraduate Clinical Performance to Monitor
        Change in the Medical School....................   23
1.2.12 Baccalaureate Preparation for Medical School:
        Does Type of Degree Make a Difference?..........   24
1.2.13 Levels of Recommendation for Students and Academic
        Performance in Medical School...................   25

2   **Demographics**   27
    2.1 Standardized Patient Assessment of Medical Student Empathy:
         Ethnicity and Gender Effects in a Multi-institutional Study   30
    2.2 Gender Segregation by Specialty During Medical School   31
    2.3 Comparing the Accuracies of Entire-Group and Subgroup Model
         to Predict NBME I Scores for Medical School Applicants   32
    2.4 African-American and White Physicians: A Comparison
         of Satisfaction with Medical Education, Professional
         Careers, and Research Activities   33
    2.5 Performance and Career Expectations of Women Medical
         Students: A Comparison with Men   34
    2.6 Gender Comparisons of Medical Students' Psychosocial
         Profiles...   35
    2.7 Gender Comparisons of Income Expectations in the USA
         at the Beginning of Medical School During the Past 28 Years   36
    2.8 Salary Inequities and Healthcare Costs   37
    2.9 Gender Comparisons of Young Physicians' Perceptions
         of Their Medical Education, Professional Life, and Practice:
         A Follow-Up Study of Jefferson Medical College Graduates   38

2.10 Gender Comparisons Prior to, During, and After Medical
School Using Two Decades of Longitudinal Data at Jefferson
Medical College 39
2.11 Change of Interest in Surgery During Medical School:
A Comparison of Men and Women 40
2.12 Prediction of Students' Performance on Licensing Examinations
Using Age, Race, Sex, Undergraduate GPAs, and MCAT Scores .. 41
2.13 A National Study of Factors Influencing Primary Care Career
Choices Among Underrepresented Minority, White,
and Asian-American Physicians 42
2.14 Performance on the NBME Part I Examination. 43
2.15 Board Certification: Associations with Physicians' Demographics
and Performances During Medical School and Residency 44
2.16 Longitudinal Comparison of the Academic Performances
of Asian-American and White Medical Students. 45

3 Medical School Evaluations 47
3.1 Preclinical 50
3.1.1 An Empirical Study of the Predictive Validity
of Number Grades in Medical School Using
Three Decades of Longitudinal Data: Implications
for a Grading System 50
3.1.2 The Fate of Medical Students with Different Levels
of Knowledge: Are the Basic Medical Sciences
Relevant to Physician Competence? 51
3.1.3 Sooner or Later? USMLE Step 1 Performance and Test
Administration Date at the End of the Second Year 52
3.1.4 Using Ratings of Resident Competence to Evaluate
NBME Examination Passing Standards. 53
3.2 Clinical. 54
3.2.1 Students' Ratings of Otolaryngology Clerkship
Activities: The Role of Residents 54
3.2.2 A Comparison of Medical Students' Self-Reported
Empathy with Simulated Patients' Assessments
of the Students' Empathy. 55
3.2.3 The Relationship Between Performance on a Medical
School's Clinical Skills Assessment and USMLE
Step 2 CS 56
3.2.4 Validity of Faculty Ratings of Students' Clinical
Competence in Core Clerkships in Relation to Scores
on Licensing Examinations and Supervisors' Ratings
in Residency. 57
3.2.5 Subtest Scores of a Comprehensive Examination of Medical
Knowledge as a Function of Retention Interval. 58
3.2.6 Evaluation of the Validity of Medical Students' Self-
Assessments of Proficiency in Clinical Simulations 59

3.2.7   Students' Gender and Examination of Patients
         in a Third-Year Family Medicine Clerkship   60
3.2.8   Evaluations of Medical Students' Clinical Experiences
         in a Family Medicine Clerkship: Differences in
         Patient Encounters by Disease Severity in Different
         Clerkship Sites................................   61
3.2.9   USMLE Step 2 Performance and Test Administration
         Date in the Fourth Year of Medical School   62
3.2.10   A Comparison of the Modified Essay Question
         and Multiple-Choice Question Formats: Their
         Relationships to Clinical Performance..................   63
3.2.11   Documenting and Comparing Medical Students' Clinical
         Experiences   64
3.2.12   Student Ratings of Clerkship Activities as a Basis
         for Curriculum Modification: A 4-Year Comparison
         of Six Departments   65
3.2.13   Identifying Students at Risk of Failing the USMLE Step 2
         Clinical Skills Examination........................   66
3.2.14   Evaluation of the Surgical Clerkship Experience
         in Affiliated Hospitals: Performance on Objective
         Examinations   67
3.2.15   Do Global Rating Forms Enable Program Directors
         to Assess the ACGME Competencies?   68
3.2.16   A Preliminary Study of the Validity of Scores
         and Pass/Fail Standards for USMLE Steps 1 and 2.......   69
3.2.17   Evaluation of the Congruence Between Students'
         Postencounter Notes and Standardized Patients'
         Checklists in a Clinical Skills Examination.............   70
3.2.18   Attendings' and Residents' Teaching Role and Students'
         Overall Rating of Clinical Clerkships   71
3.2.19   Influence of Previous Clerkship Experiences on Students'
         Satisfaction with Their Current Clerkship.............   72
3.2.20   A Correlation Study of Students' Perception of Their
         Active Role as Related to Their Clerkship Experiences ...   73

4   Postgraduate and Career   75
     4.1   Clinical Competence   79
           4.1.1   Class Ranking Models for Deans' Letters and Their
                    Psychometric Evaluation   79
           4.1.2   Further Psychometric Evaluations of a Class Ranking
                    Model as a Predictor of Graduates' Clinical Competence
                    in the First Year of Residency   80
           4.1.3   Relationship Between Performance in Medical School
                    and Postgraduate Competence........................   81

4.1.4 A Case of Mistaken Identity: Signal and Noise
in Connecting Performance Assessments Before
and After Graduation from Medical School. 82

4.1.5 What Have We Learned and Where Do We Go
from Here? 83

4.1.6 Assessment Measures in Medical School, Residency,
and Practice: The Connections. 84

4.1.7 The Role of Resident Performance Evaluation in Board
Certification 85

4.1.8 Measuring the Contribution of Medical Education
to Patient Care: A Review 86

4.1.9 Validity and Importance of Low Ratings Given to Medical
School Graduates in Noncognitive Areas 87

4.1.10 Cognitive and Noncognitive Factors in Predicting
the Clinical Performance of Medical School Graduates . . . 88

4.1.11 Is the Glass Half Full or Half Empty? A Reexamination
of the Associations Between Assessment Measures
During Medical School and Clinical Competence
After Graduation 89

4.1.12 Components of Postgraduate Competence: Analyses
of 30 Years of Longitudinal Data. 90

4.1.13 Components of Clinical Competence Ratings
of Physicians: An Empirical Approach 91

4.1.14 Conceptualization and Measurement of Clinical
Competence of Residents: A Brief Rating Form
and Its Psychometric Properties. 92

4.1.15 Relationships Between Performance in Medical
School and First Postgraduate Year 93

4.1.16 Affirmative Action and Special Consideration
Admissions to Medical Education 94

4.1.17 A Validity Study of Part III of the National Board
Examination. 95

4.2 Specialization and Professional Activities 96

4.2.1 Correlates of Young Physicians' Support for Unionization
to Maintain Professional Influence 96

4.2.2 Stability and Change of Interest in Obstetrics-
Gynecology Among Medical Students: 18 Years
of Longitudinal Data 97

4.2.3 Medical Education and Health Services Research:
The Linkage. 98

4.2.4 The Impact of Early Career Specialization on Licensing
Requirements and Related Educational Implications 99

4.2.5 The Impact of Early Specialization on the Clinical
Competence of Residents. 100

4.2.6 Should Half of All Medical School Graduates Enter
       Primary Care? Perceptions of Faculty Members
       at Jefferson Medical College 101
4.2.7 Family Medicine and Primary Care: Trends and Student
       Characteristics 102
4.2.8 Primary Care and Non-primary Care Physicians:
       A Longitudinal Study of Their Similarities,
       Differences, and Correlates Before, During,
       and After Medical School 103
4.2.9 Differences in Professional Activities, Perceptions
       of Professional Problems, and Practice Patterns
       Between Men and Women Graduates of Jefferson
       Medical College 104
4.2.10 A Program to Increase the Number of Family Physicians
       in Rural and Underserved Areas: Impact After 22 Years ... 105
4.2.11 Critical Factors for Designing Programs to Increase
       the Supply and Retention of Rural Primary
       Care Physicians 106
4.2.12 Who Is a Generalist? An Analysis of Whether Physicians
       Trained as Generalists Practice as Generalists. 107
4.2.13 A Statewide System to Track Medical Students'
       Careers: The Pennsylvania Model 108
4.2.14 Generalist Career Plans: Tracking Medical School
       Seniors Through Residency 109
4.2.15 Choice of First-Year Residency Position and Long-Term
       Generalist Career Choices 110
4.2.16 Assessment of Physicians' Interest in Primary
       Care Training/Retraining 111
4.2.17 Changing Specialties: Do Anesthesiologists
       Differ from Other Physicians? 112
4.2.18 Migration of Physicians to and from Anesthesiology 113
4.2.19 Academic Performance of Psychiatrists Compared
       to Other Specialists Before, During, and After Medical
       School 114
4.2.20 Board Certification in Obstetrics and Gynecology:
       Associations with Physicians' Demographics
       and Performances During Medical School 115
4.2.21 Performance on the NBME Part II Examination
       and Career Choice 116
4.2.22 Medical Students Who Enter General Surgery Residency
       Programs: A Follow-Up Between 1972 and 1986 117
4.2.23 Perceptions of Practice Problems Encountered by Family
       Physicians, Pediatricians, and Orthopedic Surgeons 118

4.2.24   Primary Care and Non-primary Care Physicians'
            Concerns in Practice and Perceptions of Medical
            School Curriculum............................... 119
4.2.25   Factors Associated with Changing Levels of Interest
            in Primary Care During Medical School.............. 120
4.2.26   Emergency Medicine Career Change: Associations
            with Performances in Medical School and in the First
            Postgraduate Year and with Indebtedness 121
4.2.27   The Changing Healthcare System: A Research
            Agenda for Medical Education 122
4.2.28   A National Study of the Factors Influencing Men
            and Women Physicians' Choices of Primary Care
            Specialties 123
4.2.29   A Comparison of Jefferson Medical College
            Graduates Who Chose Emergency Medicine
            with Those Who Chose Other Specialties 124
4.2.30   Factors Influencing Physicians' Decisions to Remain
            in Emergency Medicine........................... 125
4.2.31   Comparing the Academic Performances of Geriatricians
            and Other Family Physicians and Internists............. 126
4.2.32   Comparisons Among Three Types of Generalist
            Physicians: Personal Characteristics, Medical School
            Experiences, Financial Aid, and Other Factors
            Influencing Career Choice......................... 127
4.2.33   Changing Interest in Family Medicine and Students'
            Academic Performance 128
4.2.34   Physicians' Intention to Stay in or Leave Primary
            Care Specialties and Variables Associated with Such
            Intention....................................... 129
4.2.35   Factors Influencing Primary Care Physicians'
            Choice to Practice in Medically Underserved Areas...... 130
4.2.36   Factors Influencing Physicians' Choices to Practice
            in Inner-City or Rural Areas 131

5   Psychosocial Attributes................................... 133
    5.1   Effects of a Brief Curricular Intervention on Medical
            Students' Attitudes Toward People with Disabilities
            in Healthcare Settings 137
    5.2   Psychostimulant Drug Abuse and Personality Factors
            in Medical Students.............................. 138
    5.3   Volunteer Bias in Medical Education Research: An Empirical
            Study of Over Three Decades of Longitudinal Data........... 139
    5.4   Economic Diversity in Medical Education: The Relationship
            Between Students' Family Income and Academic
            Performance, Career Choice, and Student Debt 140

5.5   Characteristics of Medical Students Completing an Honors
      Program in Pathology   141
5.6   Biotechnology and Ethics in Medical Education of the New
      Millennium: Physician Roles and Responsibilities   142
5.7   Medical Students' Opinions Concerning the Healthcare
      System   143
5.8   Medical Students' Opinions on Economic Aspects
      of the Healthcare System.............................   144
5.9   Professional Attitudes and Interpersonal Relationships
      of Physicians: Are They a Problem?   145
5.10 Perception of Maternal Availability in Childhood and Selected
      Psychosocial Characteristics in Adulthood   146
5.11 Satisfaction with Early Relationships with Parents
      and Psychosocial Attributes in Adulthood: Which Parent
      Contributes More?...................................   147
5.12 Medical Students' Personal Values and Their Career
      Choices a Quarter-Century Later........................   148
5.13 Students' Personality and Ratings of Clinical Competence
      in Medical School Clerkships: A Longitudinal Study   149
5.14 Personality Assessments and Outcomes in Medical
      Education and the Practice of Medicine: AMEE Guide No. 79 ...   150
5.15 Associations Between Selected Psychosocial Attributes
      and Ratings of Physician Competence.....................   151
5.16 Physicians' Perceptions of the Changing Healthcare System:
      Comparisons by Gender and Specialties   152
5.17 Medical Student's Cognitive Appraisal of Stressful Life
      Events as Related to Personality, Physical Well-Being,
      and Academic Performance: A Longitudinal Study............   153
5.18 Career Satisfaction and Professional Accomplishments   154
5.19 Psychosocial Characteristics of Female Students in the Allied
      Health and Medical Colleges: Psychometrics of the Measures
      and Personality Profiles   155
5.20 Empathy Scores in Medical School and Ratings of Empathic
      Behavior in Residency Training 3 Years Later................   156
5.21 Can Empathy, Other Personality Attributes, and Level
      of Positive Social Influence in Medical School Identify
      Potential Leaders in Medicine?   157
5.22 A Comparison of the Personality Profiles of Internal Medicine
      Residents, Physician Role Models, and the General Population ...   158
5.23 Students' Psychosocial Characteristics as Predictors
      of Academic Performance in Medical School   159
5.24 Empathic and Sympathetic Orientations Toward Patient Care:
      Conceptualization, Measurement, and Psychometrics..........   160

5.25 Attitudes Toward Managed Care: A Brief Instrument to Measure
      Attitudes of Medical Students Toward Change in the Healthcare
      System   161
5.26 Perceptions of Medical School Seniors of the Current Changes
      in the US Healthcare System   162
5.27 Underlying Construct of Empathy, Optimism, and Burnout
      in Medical Students   163
5.28 The Devil Is in the Third Year: A Longitudinal Study
      of Erosion of Empathy in Medical School.   164
5.29 Effects of Academic and Psychosocial Predictors of Performance
      in Medical School on Coefficients of Determination   165
5.30 Personality and Specialty Interest in Medical Students.   166
5.31 The Relationship Between Grit and Selected Personality
      Measures in Medical Students   167
5.32 Predicting Peer Nominations: A Social Network Approach   168
5.33 Identifying Potential Engaging Leaders Within Medical
      Education: The Role of Positive Influence on Peers   169
5.34 How Much Do Medical Students Know About
      Physician Income?   170
5.35 Correlates of Physicians' Endorsement of the Legalization
      of Physician-Assisted Suicide   171
5.36 Peer Nominations as Related to Academic Attainment,
      Empathy, Personality, and Specialty Interest.   172
5.37 Intra- and Intercultural Comparisons of Personality
      Profiles of Medical Students in Argentina and the USA   173
5.38 Persistent Impostor Phenomenon is Associated
      with Distress in Medical Students   174
5.39 Income Expectations of First-Year Students at Jefferson Medical
      College as a Predictor of Family Practice Specialty Choice   175
5.40 Mindfulness-Based Stress Reduction Lowers Psychological
      Distress in Medical Students   176
5.41 The Income Expectations of Medical Students in the Time
      Period 1970–1980   177
5.42 Students' Certainty During Course Test-Taking
      and Performance on Clerkships and Board Exams   178

6   Professionalism   179
    6.1 Medical Students' Self-Reported Empathy and Simulated
         Patients' Assessments of Student Empathy: An Analysis
         by Gender and Ethnicity   182
    6.2 Comparisons of Nurses and Physicians on an Operational
         Measure of Empathy   183
    6.3 Change in Empathy in Medical School   184
    6.4 Enhancing and Sustaining Empathy in Medical Students   185

6.5   Patient Perceptions of Clinician's Empathy: Measurement
       and Psychometrics   186
6.6   Empathy of Medical Students and Compassionate Care
       for Dying Patients: An Assessment of "No One Dies Alone"
       Program   187
6.7   Empathy: An NP/MD Comparison   188
6.8   Attitudes Toward Physician-Nurse Alliance: Comparisons
       of Medical and Nursing Students.   189
6.9   Psychometric Properties of an Attitude Scale Measuring
       Physician-Nurse Collaboration   190
6.10   An Instrument for Measuring Pharmacist and Physician Attitudes
       Toward Collaboration: Preliminary Psychometric Data   191
6.11   Eleven Years of Data on the Jefferson Scale of Empathy-Medical
       Student Version (JSE-S): Proxy Norm Data and Tentative
       Cutoff Scores   192
6.12   Letter to the Editor: In Reply to Quinn and Zelenski   193
6.13   What Matters More About the Interpersonal Reactivity Index
       and the Jefferson Scale of Empathy? Their Underlying
       Constructs or Their Relationships with Pertinent Measures
       of Clinical Competence and Patient Outcomes   194
6.14   Physician Empathy in Medical Education and Practice:
       Experience with the Jefferson Scale of Physician Empathy   195
6.15   Empathy in Medical Students as Related to Academic
       Performance, Clinical Competence, and Gender.   196
6.16   Comparisons of American, Israeli, Italian, and Mexican
       Physicians and Nurses on the Total and Factor Scores
       of the Jefferson Scale of Attitudes Toward Physician-Nurse
       Collaborative Relationships.   197
6.17   The Jefferson Scale of Physician Empathy: Further
       Psychometric Data and Differences by Gender and Specialty
       at Item Level   198
6.18   Physician Empathy: Definition, Components, Measurement,
       and Relationship to Gender and Specialty.   199
6.19   Rebuttals to Critics of Studies of the Decline of Empathy   200
6.20   Developing an Instrument to Measure Attitudes Toward Nurses:
       Preliminary Psychometric Findings.   201
6.21   Exploration and Confirmation of the Latent Variable
       Structure of the Jefferson Scale of Empathy   202
6.22   The Jefferson Scale of Empathy (JSE): An Update.   203
6.23   Editorial: Empathy and Health Care Quality.   204
6.24   Empathy in Medical Education and Patient Care   205
6.25   Relationships Between Scores of the Jefferson Scale
       of Physician Empathy (JSPE) and the Interpersonal
       Reactivity Index (IRI)   206

6.26 The Jefferson Scale of Physician Empathy: Development
      and Preliminary Psychometric Data.   207
6.27 An Empirical Study of Decline in Empathy in Medical School . . .   208
6.28 Attitudes Toward Physician-Nurse Collaboration:
      A Cross-cultural Study of Male and Female Physicians
      and Nurses in the USA and Mexico.   209
6.29 An Operational Measure of Physician Lifelong Learning: Its
      Development, Components, and Preliminary Psychometric Data. .   210
6.30 Psychometrics of the Scale of Attitudes Toward
      Physician-Pharmacist Collaboration: A Study with Medical
      Students   211
6.31 Measurement and Correlates of Physicians' Lifelong Learning . . .   212
6.32 Physician Lifelong Learning: Conceptualization,
      Measurement, and Correlates in Full-Time Clinicians
      and Academic Clinicians   213
6.33 Assessing Physicians' Orientation Toward Lifelong Learning   214
6.34 The Jefferson Scale of Attitudes Toward Interprofessional
      Collaboration (JEFFSATIC): Development and Multi-institution
      Psychometric Data.   215
6.35 Empathy in Medical Students as Related to Specialty Interest,
      Personality, and Perceptions of Mother and Father   216
6.36 Enhancing Student Empathetic Engagement, History-Taking,
      and Communication Skills During Electronic Medical
      Record Use in Patient Care   217
6.37 Assessment of Empathy in Different Years of Internal
      Medicine Training   218
6.38 Evaluating the Relationship Between Participation
      in Student-Run Free Clinics and Changes in Empathy
      in Medical Students   219
6.39 Measuring Professionalism: A Review of Studies with
      Instruments Reported in the Literature Between 1982 and 2002 . .   220
6.40 Linguistic Analysis of Empathy in Medical School Admission
      Essays.   221

7   Miscellaneous.   223
7.1   Medical Education, Social Accountability, and Patient
      Outcomes   225
7.2   AM Last Page: The Jefferson Longitudinal Study of Medical
      Education   226
7.3   Viewpoint: Guiding Medical Students Toward Empathetic
      Patient Care   228
7.4   Jefferson Medical College Longitudinal Study: A Prototype
      for Evaluation of Changes   229
7.5   Creating a Longitudinal Database in Medical Education:
      Perspectives from the Pioneers   230

7.6   Disciplinary Action by Medical Boards and Prior Behavior
      in Medical School   231
7.7   The Jefferson Longitudinal Study of Medical Education:
      Five Decades of Outcome Assessment   232

Bibliography   233

Name Index   247

Subject Index..   251

About the Authors

Joseph S. Gonnella, MD received his BA from Dartmouth College (summa cum laude) and his MD from Harvard Medical School. He has been awarded the Commendatore dell'Ordine della Stella della Solidarieta Italiana; the Grande Ufficiale by the President of the Italian Republic; the Dongbaeg Medal by the President of Korea; the Presidential Medal by Dartmouth College; and the Presidential Citation by Thomas Jefferson University. He has received honorary degrees from the University of Chieti, Italy. Soonchunhyang University, Korea; International Medical University of Malaysia; and the University of Minho, Portugal. He has also received the Abraham Flexner Award from the Association of American Medical Colleges and the Strittmatter Award from the Philadelphia County Medical Society. Sidney Kimmel Medical College, Thomas Jefferson University, Philadelphia, PA, USA

Clara A. Callahan, MD received her BA degree in anthropology from Wayne State University. She attended the Medical College of Pennsylvania, where she did 2 years of her pediatric residency before moving to Jefferson to complete her last year of residency training. Dr. Callahan was appointed to the Pediatrics faculty in 1982 and joined the Dean's Staff of the Medical College in 1987. After initially working in Student Affairs, she became the Dean for Admissions in 1999. Given Dr. Callahan's long-time involvement with medical students, it is not surprising that much of her research centers on the performance of students in medical school and beyond. Sidney Kimmel Medical College, Thomas Jefferson University, Philadelphia, PA, USA

J. Jon Veloski, MS career began in 1970 at Thomas Jefferson University in information technology, and he moved to the medical college in 1973 to develop the database of the Jefferson Longitudinal Study. During the past 50 years, he has published over 150 scientific research papers in peer-reviewed journals including the *New England Journal of Medicine*, the *Journal of the American Medical Association*, *Academic Medicine*, and other US and international journals. While the majority were based on data in the Jefferson Longitudinal Study reported herein, many used new data sets constructed with funding from the U.S. Health Resources and Services Administration, the Accreditation Council on Graduate Medical Education, the American Board of Family Medicine, and the American Board of Internal Medicine. He completed his BS at Drexel University and his MS and doctoral coursework in measurement, evaluation, and research at the University of Pennsylvania. Sidney Kimmel Medical College, Thomas Jefferson University, Philadelphia, PA, USA

Jennifer DeSantis, MEd received her M.Ed. from Stanford University and her BA from Vassar College. Her work focuses on empathy in medical education and health care at Jefferson University as well as nationally and internationally in collaboration with other institutions. Her background is in educational research and psychological sciences. Sidney Kimmel Medical College, Thomas Jefferson University, Philadelphia, PA, USA

Mohammadreza Hojat, PhD received his BA degree in educational psychology from Pahlavi University (currently University of Shiraz), his MA degree in psychology from the University of Tehran, and his Ph.D. in psychological services from the University of Pennsylvania. Dr. Hojat is a licensed psychologist and has published more than 270 articles in peer-reviewed journals and 13 book chapters on educational, psychological, and social issues. Dr. Hojat has developed ten psychometrically sound instruments (including the well-known *Jefferson Scale of Empathy*) for the assessment of health professions education and patient outcomes. Dr. Hojat's research on measurement, development, erosion, enhancement, and correlates of empathy in health professions education and patient care has received broad media coverage, featured in the *New York Times*, *Wall Street Journal*, *Philadelphia Inquirer*, the *National Public Radio*, and television program segments. Dr. Hojat has served as a co-editor of two books: *Loneliness: Theory, Research, and Applications* (Sage Publications, 1987) and *Assessment Measures in Medical School, Residency, and Practice: The Connections* (Springer, 1993). The second edition of his seminal book "*Empathy in Health Professions Education and Patient Care*" was published in 2016 (Springer International Publishing). Sidney Kimmel Medical College, Thomas Jefferson University, Philadelphia, PA, USA

Chapter 1
Admissions

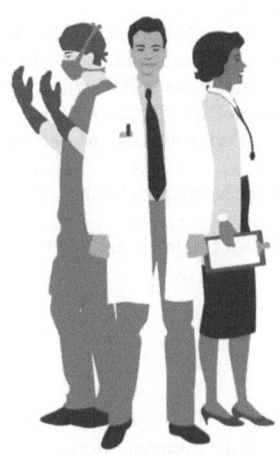

Contents

1.1		Standardized Tests.	4
	1.1.1	The Predictive Validity of Three Versions of the MCAT in Relation to Performance in Medical School, Residency, and Licensing Examinations: A Longitudinal Study of 36 Classes of Jefferson Medical College.	4
	1.1.2	Science, Verbal, or Quantitative Skills: Which Is the Most Important Predictor of Physician Competence?.	5
	1.1.3	A Validity Study of the Writing Sample Section of the Medical College Admission Test.	6
	1.1.4	Predictive Validity of the MCAT for Students with Two Sets of Scores.	7
	1.1.5	Delays in Completing Medical School: Predictors and Outcomes.	8
	1.1.6	The Overall Validity of the New MCAT.	9
	1.1.7	Long-Range Predictive and Differential Validities of the Scholastic Aptitude Test in Medical School.	10
	1.1.8	Predictive Validity of the MCAT as a Function of Undergraduate Institutions.	11
	1.1.9	The Relationship Between MCAT Science Subtest Scores and Performance in Medical School: The Impact of the Undergraduate Institution.	12
1.2		Academic Preparation.	13
	1.2.1	Reexamination of Relationships Between Students' Undergraduate Majors, Medical School Performances, and Career Plans at Jefferson Medical College.	13
	1.2.2	The Jefferson-Penn State BS-MD Program: A 26-Year Experience.	14
	1.2.3	Evaluation of an Enrichment Program for Entering Medical Students Predicted to Be in Need of Academic Preparation.	15
	1.2.4	Preparing for the MD: How Long, at What Cost, and with What Outcomes?.	16
	1.2.5	Premedical Training, Personal Characteristics, and Performance in Medical School.	17

1.2.6   Assessments of Empathy in Medical School Admissions: What Additional
        Evidence Is Needed?...   18
1.2.7   Postbaccalaureate Preparation and Performance in Medical School.............   19
1.2.8   A Program to Recruit and Educate Medical Students to Practice Family
        Medicine in Underserved Areas..   20
1.2.9   Evaluation of a Selective Medical School Admission Policy to Increase the
        Number of Family Physicians in Rural and Underserved Areas.................   21
1.2.10 Demographic, Educational, and Economic Factors Related to Recruitment
        and Retention of Physicians in Rural Pennsylvania.............................   22
1.2.11 Using Postgraduate Clinical Performance to Monitor Change in the Medical
        School...   23
1.2.12 Baccalaureate Preparation for Medical School: Does Type of Degree Make
        a Difference?...   24
1.2.13 Levels of Recommendation for Students and Academic Performance
        in Medical School...   25

Abstract

Selecting applicants to medical school to become competent physicians is a challenging issue for medical schools. This chapter includes studies addressing which standardized test scores could predict academic and clinical performances in medical school, and whether preferential admission criteria can be of help in achieving the goals of targeted medical education programs. The chapter includes two subsections.

Standardized Tests (MCAT and SAT)
- Findings generally suggest that MCAT science subtest scores of its three versions (pre-1978, 1987–1991, and post-1991) could significantly predict performance in the preclinical phase of medical school education.
- Scores on the Writing Sample of the MCAT were significantly associated with indicators of clinical competence in medical school.
- Delayed graduation for academic reasons was significantly associated with the Science and Reading MCAT subtest scores.
- Findings for students with repeated MCAT scores suggested that an average of repeated sets of MCAT scores was the best predictor of medical school performance, followed by sets of early, lower, higher, and later MCAT scores.
- Scores on the SAT (taken in high school) were significantly associated with performance measures in medical school.

Academic Preparation
- Preferentially selected applicants (per residential area, backgrounds, and career plans) were significantly more likely to enter family medicine residency programs, and become family physicians, compared to their classmates.
- Comparisons of graduates of an accelerated program to obtain combined BS and MD degrees in 5–6 years after high school with a matched group of their classmates confirmed that it is feasible to obtain an MD degree in a shorter time and at lower cost without compromising educational outcomes and professional competence.

Keywords Baccalaureate preparation · Career plan · Combined BS-MD degree program · Delayed graduation · Demographics · Economic factor · Empathy score in admission decisions · Letters of recommendation · Medical College Admission Test (MCAT) · National Board Medical Examinations · Penn State-Jefferson Accelerated Program · Postbaccalaureate preparation · Predictive validity of admission measures · Preferential selection · Repeated MCAT · Retention · Scholastic Aptitude Test (SAT) · Selection of applicants · Undergraduate grade point average · Undergraduate institutions · Undergraduate major · Underserved areas · Verbal skills

1.1   Standardized Tests

1.1.1   The Predictive Validity of Three Versions of the MCAT in Relation to Performance in Medical School, Residency, and Licensing Examinations: A Longitudinal Study of 36 Classes of Jefferson Medical College

Clara A. Callahan, Mohammadreza Hojat, Jon Veloski, James B. Erdmann, and Joseph S. Gonnella

Purpose: The Medical College Admission Test (MCAT) has undergone several revisions for content and validity since its inception. With another comprehensive review pending, this study examines changes in the predictive validity of the MCAT's three recent versions.

Method: Study participants were 7859 matriculants in 36 classes entering Jefferson Medical College between 1970 and 2005; 1728 took the pre-1978 version of the MCAT; 3032 took the 1978–1991 version; and 3099 took the post-1991 version. MCAT subtest scores were the predictors, and performance in medical school, attrition, scores on the medical licensing examinations, and ratings of clinical competence in the first year of residency were the criterion measures.

Results: No significant improvement in validity coefficients was observed for performance in medical school or residency. Validity coefficients for all three versions of the MCAT in predicting Part I/Step 1 remained stable (in the mid-0.40s, $p < 0.01$). A systematic decline was observed in the validity coefficients of the MCAT versions in predicting Part II/Step 2. It started at 0.47 for the pre-1978 version, decreased to between 0.42 and 0.40 for the 1978–1991 versions, and to 0.37 for the post-1991 version. Validity coefficients for the MCAT versions in predicting Part III/Step 3 remained near 0.30. These were generally higher for women than men.

Conclusions: Although the findings support the short- and long-term predictive validity of the MCAT, opportunities to strengthen it remain. Subsequent revisions should increase the test's ability to predict performance on the United States Medical Licensing Examination Step 2 and must minimize the differential validity for gender.

Academic Medicine, 2010, *85*(6), 980–987. https://doi.org/10.1097/ACM.0b013e3181cece3d

1.1.2   *Science, Verbal, or Quantitative Skills: Which Is the Most Important Predictor of Physician Competence?*

Karen Glaser, Mohammadreza Hojat, J. Jon Veloski, Robert S. Blacklow, and Carla E. Goepp

The relative importance of medical school applicants' science problem-solving, reading, and quantitative skills as measured by the Medical College Admission Test (MCAT) was studied in predicting competence measured by the three parts of the National Board of Examinations (NBE). Subjects were 1628 physicians graduated from Jefferson Medical College between 1978 and 1985. The results of bivariate and multiple correlations indicated that scores on the science problems subtest were better predictors of the basic science component of physician education (Part I scores of the NBE) than the reading scores. Both the science problems and reading skills predicted clinical science scores equally well (Part II scores of the NBE). Reading skills scores contributed more than the science problems subtest in predicting scores on an examination of patient management skills (Part III of the NBE). Scores of the quantitative skills subtest did not contribute to any prediction. These findings suggest that the great emphasis placed by medical school admissions committees on science problem-solving scores of the MCAT is justifiable if performance in the basic science component of medical education is taken as the target outcome measure. However, if clinical skills in medical practice are taken as a target criterion, then at least equal emphasis should be placed on reading skills scores of the MCAT. It is discussed that there may be a potential value in improving the reading skills of medical school students in order to enhance their clinical and patient management competence. Implications of these findings in support of the new MCAT are discussed.

Educational and Psychological Measurement, 1992, *52*(2), 395–405.

1.1.3   A Validity Study of the Writing Sample Section of the Medical College Admission Test

Mohammadreza Hojat, James B. Erdmann, J. Jon Veloski, Thomas J. Nasca, Clara A. Callahan, Ellen Julian, and Jeremy Peck

Problem Statement and Background: This study examined the validity of the Writing Sample section of the current Medical College Admission Test (MCAT) and tested the hypothesis that the Writing Sample scores would be more closely associated with indicators of clinical competence than with basic sciences achievement measures.

Method: In a longitudinal design, 1776 matriculants at Jefferson Medical College between 1992 and 1999 were studied. Top, middle, and bottom scorers on the Writing Sample were compared on measures of performance in the basic and clinical sciences during medical school and beyond.

Results: The research hypothesis was supported. Scores on the Writing Sample were significantly associated with indicators of clinical competence, even when statistical adjustments were made for score differences in other sections of the MCAT.

Conclusions: Findings support the validity of the Writing Sample from a number of perspectives.

Academic Medicine, 2000, *75* (October Supplement), S25–S27. https://journals. lww.com/academicmedicine/Fulltext/2000/10001/A_Validity_Study_of_the_ Writing_Sample_Section_of.8.aspx

1.1.4   Predictive Validity of the MCAT for Students with Two Sets of Scores

Mohammadreza Hojat, J. Jon Veloski, and Carter Zeleznik

This study addresses the question of which set of scores for those students who retake the Medical College Admission Test (MCAT) yields a better predictive validity. The sample comprised of 304 students who retook the MCAT prior to entering Jefferson Medical College between 1978 and 1981. Five sets of MCAT scores were considered as predictors in the study: earlier, later, higher, and lower sets of MCAT scores and the average of the earlier and later scores for each MCAT subtest. Twenty-five criteria were used, including grades earned in the freshman and sophomore years and scores on the subtests of Part I and Part II of the examinations of the National Board of Medical Examiners. Correlational techniques, such as bivariate and multiple correlation analyses and canonical correlation followed by redundancy analysis, were utilized. The magnitude of redundancy indices indicated that the set of MCAT scores in which the earlier and later scores were averaged was the best predictor, followed by the earlier, lower, higher, and later sets of MCAT scores. The implications of these findings for the admission process and for validity studies are discussed.

Journal of Medical Education, 1985, *60,* 911–918. https://doi. org/10.1097/00001888-198512000-00002

1.1.5   Delays in Completing Medical School: Predictors and Outcomes

Leonard M. Rosenfeld, Mohammadreza Hojat, J. Jon Veloski, Robert S. Blacklow, and Carla E. Goepp

This study addresses whether delayed graduation due to academic difficulties in the early years of medical school can be predicted early and whether such difficulties are likely to be manifested in later clinical clerkships and residency. A group of 103 graduates who entered Jefferson Medical College between 1970 and 1984 and who required more than 4 years to complete their studies due to academic difficulties were compared with a random sample of 120 on-time graduates. Statistically significant differences were observed between delayed and on-time graduates on measures of performance before, during, and after medical school in the favor of on-time graduates. Scores of 8 on the Medical College Admission Test (MCAT) and an undergraduate science grade-point average of 3.25 were found to be pivotal points below which the likelihood of delayed graduation was higher than the likelihood of on-time graduation. Discriminant analysis indicated that 76% of delayed and on-time graduates could correctly be classified into their respective groups by using admission variables. These findings suggest that predictors of delayed graduation can be detected early in medical school and that the academic difficulties that resulted in delayed graduation are likely to continue through postgraduate training. Recognition of the chronic nature of these differences should alert medical schools to monitor carefully the performance of students who are delayed because of academic difficulties and provide appropriate support on a continuing basis to enhance performance.

Teaching and Learning in Medicine, 1992, *4*(3), 162–167. https://www.tandfonline.com/doi/abs/10.1080/10401339209539556

1.1.6   The Overall Validity of the New MCAT

J. Jon Veloski, Mohammadreza Hojat, and Carter Zeleznik

This study was designed to provide information about the overall relationship(s) between the new MCAT scales and selected measures of academic performance. The study sample comprised of data on 213 students who matriculated at Jefferson Medical College in 1978. The data included, in addition to the new MCAT scales, course grades obtained in the freshman and sophomore years and scores achieved on Part I of the National Board of Examinations. Three statistical correlation techniques were used in analyzing the data: simple, multiple, and canonical correlation.

Approximately 46% of the variance in the new MCAT linear composites and Part I of the NBME were accounted for in the canonical correlations of Rc1 = 0.61 and Rc2 = 0.38. Loadings of the canonical components indicated that the new MCAT scales measure performance in the science problems, chemistry, and physics as well as a verbally related dimension. Excluding the science problems, biology, chemistry, and physics from the global analysis did not change significantly the overall indices of relationships. The findings of this study support the validity of the new MCAT as an overall predictive measure of performance in the freshman and sophomore years of medical school.

Proceedings of the Twentieth Annual Conference on Research in Medical Education, Washington, DC. November 1981, 129–134. https://pubmed.ncbi.nlm.nih. gov/7347515/
This abstract was written by the book editors.

1.1.7   Long-Range Predictive and Differential Validities
of the Scholastic Aptitude Test in Medical School

Carter Zeleznik, Mohammadreza Hojat, and J. Jon Veloski

This study was designed to determine the predictive and differential validity of the Scholastic Aptitude Test (SAT). Data derived from a longitudinal study of 1284 students who entered Jefferson Medical College in the years 1965 through 1974 were analyzed. The students were divided into four groups according to their earned scores on the verbal and quantitative scales of the SAT.

When analysis of variance was applied to the data, a significant relationship was found between SAT scores and academic achievement levels in medical school. Those students who scored high on the SAT achieved higher grades (scores) on the standardized measures of achievement and those who scored low on the SAT scored lower on the standardized measures. The validity of the SAT as a predictor of future academic performance was supported by our findings.

Educational and Psychological Measurement, 1983, *43*, 223–232.
    Copyright© 1983. Sage Publishing. https://doi.org/10.1177/001316448304300129

1.1.8 Predictive Validity of the MCAT as a Function of Undergraduate Institutions

Carter Zeleznik, Mohammadreza Hojat, and J. Jon Veloski

The question of whether the predictive ability of the Medical College Admission Test (MCAT) differed for students from different undergraduate institutions was addressed in this study. Two groups of students were studied: group 1 comprised 1859 students who entered Jefferson Medical College between 1964 and 1977, and group 2 consisted of 999 students who entered the college between 1978 and 1982. Ten undergraduate institutions with at least 20 matriculants in each group were selected for analysis. Group 1 students had taken the old version and group 2 the new version of the MCAT. Scores on the science subtest of the old MCAT were used as the predictor for group 1, and scores on the science problems subtest of the new MCAT were used as the predictor for group 2. First-year and second-year medical school grade-point averages and total scores on the Part I and Part II examinations of the National Board of Medical Examiners were the performance measures used. Validity coefficients were derived of the predictive value of the MCAT scores at each of the 10 undergraduate institutions. Striking differences were found in validity coefficients among these institutions. These differences raise questions about the predictive validity of the MCAT when scores for different undergraduate institutions are combined in deriving the coefficients. Possible explanations, implications for admission decisions and validity studies, and limitations of these findings are discussed.

Journal of Medical Education, 1987, *62,* 163–169. https://doi.org/10.1097/00001888-198703000-00003
   Reprinted in *The Advisor,* 1987, *7*(3), 1–4.

1.1.9 The Relationship Between MCAT Science Subtest Scores and Performance in Medical School: The Impact of the Undergraduate Institution

Carter Zeleznik, J. Jon Veloski, Samuel Conly Jr., and Mohammadreza Hojat

This study was designed to examine the validity of the Medical College Admission Test (MCAT) science subtest as a predictor of student performance in medical school. Consideration was given to the undergraduate college attended by each student. Jefferson Medical College, in association with eight undergraduate institutions from which it accepts a large number of students, established a cooperative longitudinal study. Summary statistics were computed on mean MCAT scores, National Board of Examination scores, and other performance measures. Data were collected on the students entering medical schools in the years 1965 through 1977, using the "old MCAT." Results obtained in this study indicated considerable variations in correlations between MCAT science scores and measures of medical school performances. The findings suggested that, based on the MCAT science scores and the undergraduate institution attended by the individual, it is possible to predict the degree of a student's success in some areas of medical school. It was concluded that the MCAT could be considered not a "nationally standardized" test but one requiring standardization in relation to many factors.

Proceedings of the Nineteenth Annual Conference on Research in Medical Education, Washington, DC. October 1980, 257–262.
    This abstract was written by the book editors.

1.2   Academic Preparation

1.2.1   Reexamination of Relationships Between Students' Undergraduate Majors, Medical School Performances, and Career Plans at Jefferson Medical College

Hidemichi Ashikawa, Mohammadreza Hojat, Carter Zeleznik,
and Joseph S. Gonnella

A reexamination of the possible relationships between medical students' undergraduate academic majors and their medical school performances and career plans seems appropriate, given the continuing changes in the characteristics of the medical school applicant pool in the last several years. This study investigated these relationships by comparing cognitive and noncognitive characteristics of medical students who had different undergraduate majors. The study sample consisted of 812 students who entered Jefferson Medical College between 1985 and 1988. They were classified into six categories based on their undergraduate majors: biological, chemical and physical, social and behavioral, other sciences, humanities and arts, and indeterminate majors. Results indicated that performances in the basic science component of medical education were about the same for students with different undergraduate majors. The groups had similar rates of delayed graduation, but the attrition rate was highest for students who had majored in humanities and arts. The students in undergraduate disciplines traditionally oriented toward medicine (biological, physical, and chemical sciences) were younger and had made the decision to become a physician at earlier ages than had their counterparts with undergraduate majors in social sciences and humanities. Also, the groups differed with regard to their estimates of their future incomes and plans for professional activities after graduation. Similarities concerning the students' preferred professional activities were also noticed among the groups.

Academic Medicine, 1991, *66*, 458–464. https://doi.org/10.1097/00001888-199108000-00009

1.2.2   The Jefferson-Penn State BS-MD Program:
A 26-Year Experience

Clara A. Callahan, J. Jon Veloski, Gang Xu, Mohammadreza Hojat,
Carter Zeleznik, and Joseph S. Gonnella

Since the 1960s a number of physicians have been completing both their baccalaureate and their MD degrees in 6 or fewer years. In this longitudinal study the authors track the academic performances, clinical ratings, and career follow-up data of 659 students in one of these accelerated programs, the Jefferson Medical College-Pennsylvania State University BS-MD program, from entering years 1964 through 1989. The medical school performances, clinical performances in residencies, and rates of board certification and faculty appointment of the accelerated students were compared favorably with those of a control group of medical students with similar high school credentials who had followed a 4-year baccalaureate program. The authors conclude that a carefully chosen group of students can achieve high academic standards in an accelerated medical school program, graduate as younger physicians able to perform well in postgraduate training, and go on to highly productive careers in medicine.

Academic Medicine, 1992, *67*(11), 792–797. https://doi.org/10.1097/00001888-199211000-00019
    Reprinted (in Chinese) in *International Medicine*, 1993, *3*, 137–183.

1.2.3 Evaluation of an Enrichment Program for Entering Medical Students Predicted to Be in Need of Academic Preparation

Karen Glaser, Mohammadreza Hojat, and Clara A. Callahan

This study was designed to assess a prematriculation enrichment program for incoming matriculates who were predicted to need academic preparations prior to starting medical school education. Research participants included 585 students who entered Jefferson Medical College between 1988 and 1990. They were grouped into the following three categories: (1) those who were invited and subsequently completed the program ($n = 70$); (2) those who were invited but declined the invitation ($n = 27$); and (3) those who were not at risk of failing, and thus were not invited to participate in the enrichment program ($n = 488$). Statistical analyses showed that those who were invited and participated in the program were older than others ($p < 0.01$). The three groups differed significantly on the first-year GPAs ($p < 0.01$) with the highest mean GPAs obtained by those who were not invited to participate. Similar pattern of findings was observed among the second-year GPAs, in the third-year six core clerkship objective examinations, and in Steps 1 and Step 2 of medical licensing examinations. No significant differences were observed among the three groups on the ratings of clinical competence given in third-year core clerkships. Participants of the enrichment program expressed satisfaction for the opportunity given to them to be better prepared for medical school education.

Education for Health, 1996, 9, 221–228.
This abstract was written by the book editors.

1.2.4   Preparing for the MD: How Long, at What Cost, and with What Outcomes?

Joseph S. Gonnella, Clara A. Callahan, James B. Erdmann, J. Jon Veloski, Niusha Jafari, Ronald A. Markle, and Mohammadreza Hojat

Purpose: To assess educational and professional outcomes of an accelerated combined Bachelor of Science-Doctor of Medicine (BS-MD) program using data collected from 1968 through 2018.

Method: Participants of this longitudinal study included 2235 students who entered medical school between 1968 and 2014: 1134 in the accelerated program and 1101 in the regular curriculum (control group)—matched by year of entrance to medical school, gender, and Medical College Admission Test (MCAT) scores. Outcome measures included performance on medical licensing examinations, academic progress, satisfaction with medical school, educational debt, first-year residency program directors' ratings on clinical competence, specialty choice, board certification, and faculty appointments.

Results: The authors found no practically important differences between students in the accelerated program and those in the control group on licensing examination performance, academic progress, specialty choice, board certification, and faculty appointments. Accelerated students had lower mean educational debt ($p < 0.01$, effect sizes = 0.81 and 0.45 for, respectively, their baccalaureate debt and medical school debt), lower satisfaction with their second year ($p < 0.01$, effect size = 0.21) of medical school, and lower global satisfaction with their medical school education ($p < 0.01$, effect size = 0.35). Residency program directors' ratings in six postgraduate competency areas showed no practically important differences between the students in the accelerated program and those in the control group. The proportion of Asian students was higher among program participants ($p < 0.01$, effect size = 0.43).

Conclusions: Students in the accelerated program earned BS and MD degrees at a faster pace and pursued careers that were comparable to students in a matched control who were in a regular MD program. Findings indicate that shortening the length of medical education does not compromise educational and professional outcomes.

Academic Medicine, 2021, *96*(1),101–107.   https://doi.org/10.1097/ACM.0000000000003298

1.2.5   Premedical Training, Personal Characteristics, and Performance in Medical School

Mary W. Herman and J. Jon Veloski

The study compares attrition rates and clinical competence levels of medical students with variations in premedical training, age, and sex to determine the risks attached. No differences were found in levels of clinical competence, although groups varied in average science scores on the Medical College Admission Test (MCAT). Students with nonscience undergraduate majors scored lower on this test than science majors. Younger women had relatively high attrition rates but high performance on the MCAT science subtest and medical school science courses. While the study shows that students who are older or younger than average may have more problems that are not strictly academic, no relationships were found between premedical training and clinical competence. It was concluded that all groups in the study were adequately prepared in the basic sciences for medical school. The risk of producing physicians who are not clinically competent would not be increased by accepting students with lower science scores.

Medical   Education,   1981,   *15*,   363–367.   https://doi.org/10.1111/j.1365-2923.1981.tb02415.x

1.2.6   Assessments of Empathy in Medical School Admissions: What Additional Evidence Is Needed?

Mohammadreza Hojat

This editorial is based on a presentation at a symposium on the theme of Examining the Evidence with Regard to Character, Personality, and Values in Medical School Selection, sponsored by the Association for the Study of Medical Education (ASME). We presented evidence to refute the argument against using personality assessments in admission decisions. Because of our extensive research on the topic of empathy in medical education and patient care, we placed emphasis on credibility of evidence for using assessments of empathy in the selection of applicants to medical schools. The notion that personality is a contributing factor to academic achievement, clinical competence, career choice, and professional behavior implies that personality should be considered not only as a pertinent measure for the assessment of professional development of doctors in training, but as an additional requirement for the admission of qualified applicants to medical schools. The choice of pertinent personality attributes should be based on the following three requirements: conceptual relevancy, availability of psychometrically sound measuring instruments, and empirical link to clinical competence and patient outcomes. Empathy was described as a pertinent personality attribute that seems germane to clinical competence and an essential element of professionalism in medicine. Also, there exists a psychometrically sound instrument, the Jefferson Scale of Empathy (JSE), which was specifically developed to measure empathy in the context of medical education and patient care with extensive psychometric support. In addition, significant associations have been reported between scores of the JSE and measures of clinical competence and patient outcomes. This is the most crucial requirement in support of the credibility of empathy assessment as a supplementary admission requirement. Medical schools are socially accountable to select "qualified" applicants with the best potential to become "caring physicians" not just those who can successfully pass examinations of recalling factual knowledge. The notion of social accountability in medical school admissions could lead to a potentially new legal challenge in the future for medical schools. To avoid such legal challenges, to render more optimal care, to regain reputation of the profession of medicine, and to reclaim compassionate image of doctors, bold actions must be taken to break free from unverified assumptions, unfounded notions, and sociopolitical considerations.

International Journal of Medical Education, 2014, 5, 7–10. https://doi.org/10.5116/ijme.52b7.5294

1.2.7 Postbaccalaureate Preparation and Performance in Medical School

Mohammadreza Hojat, Robert S. Blacklow, Mary R. Robeson, J. Jon Veloski, and Bette D. Borenstein

The question whether postbaccalaureate preparation before matriculation in medical school contributes to medical students' performance was addressed by this study. A total of 610 (91%) of the students who entered Jefferson Medical College between 1985 and 1987 were the study sample. Fifty-eight of these students had taken nondegree undergraduate premedical courses and 15 had taken nondegree graduate courses. Fourteen students held graduate degrees and 60 students had some combination of the aforementioned types of postbaccalaureate preparations. The other 463 students had not taken postbaccalaureate courses. Grades received in medical school courses such as anatomy, biochemistry, mechanisms of disease, physiology, microbiology, pathology, and pharmacology, as well as total scores on Part I of the National Board of Medical Examiners' examination, were selected as performance variables.

Statistical analyses showed that the students who had taken nondegree postbaccalaureate courses had lower undergraduate grade-point averages than those without such courses and received lower grades on some measures of performance in medical school. The students with such additional academic backgrounds were also older than an average medical student. When adjustments were made for undergraduate grade-point averages by applying analysis of covariance, the observed differences that favored the group without postbaccalaureate preparation either became nonsignificant or favored those with such preparation. The differences favoring those without postbaccalaureate preparation could be accounted for mostly by these students' higher undergraduate grade-point averages and younger ages. Implications for admission decisions with regard to the changing applicant pool are discussed.

Academic Medicine, 1990, *65*, 388–391. https://journals.lww.com/academicmedicine/Abstract/1990/06000/Postbaccalaureate_preparation_and_performance_in.7.aspx

Also in *Proceedings of the Twenty-seventh Annual Conference on Research in Medical Education.* Chicago, IL. November 1988, 310–315.

1.2.8 A Program to Recruit and Educate Medical Students to Practice Family Medicine in Underserved Areas

Howard K. Rabinowitz

In an attempt to address the problem of physician maldistribution, Jefferson Medical College initiated the Physician Shortage Area Program (PSAP) in 1974, a special admission program that preferentially selects applicants who intend to practice family medicine in physician shortage areas in Pennsylvania. Forty-seven students in four classes have been graduated from the program. Evaluation of these students during medical school shows that their academic performance has been similar to that of their classmates. Follow-up evaluation indicates that PSAP graduates are five times as likely as their peers (non-PSAP) to enter a family medicine residency program during the first postgraduate year (62% versus 12%), and almost twice as likely to enter family medicine as a comparable group of non-PSAP students who originally entered Jefferson with plans of becoming a family physician (62% versus 33%).

Reproduced with permission from *Journal of the American Medical Association*, 1983, *249*(8), 1038–1041.

1.2.9 Evaluation of a Selective Medical School Admission Policy to Increase the Number of Family Physicians in Rural and Underserved Areas

Howard K. Rabinowitz

The Physician Shortage Area Program (PSAP) at Jefferson Medical College preferentially admits medical school applicants who grew up in rural areas or small towns, and who also plan to practice the specialty of family medicine in rural and underserved areas. Evaluation of graduates from the first eight classes (1978–1985) showed that PSAP graduates performed slightly less well than their non-PSAP peers during medical school, although the attrition rate during medical school and performance during postgraduate training was similar in both groups. Graduates from the first four classes (1978–1981) were tracked into their practice location, and the results showed that the PSAP graduates were almost five times as likely as their peers (59.6% vs. 12.6%, $P < 0.001$) to practice family medicine, and three times as likely to practice in rural areas (37.8–42.2% (depending on the definition of rural) vs. 10.0–11.8%, $P < 0.001$). They were similarly 2–4 times more likely to practice in an area with a physician shortage (26.7–40.0% vs. 9.2–11.2%, $P < 0.01$). PSAP graduates were 7–10 times more likely than non-PSAP graduates to have combined a career in family medicine with practice in a rural or underserved area (24.4–31.1% vs. 3.1–3.9%, $P < 0.001$). These results show that a medical school admission program can have an important impact on increasing the supply of family physicians in rural and underserved areas.

The New England Journal of Medicine, 319, 480–486.

This abstract was written by the book editors.

1.2.10   Demographic, Educational, and Economic Factors Related to Recruitment and Retention of Physicians in Rural Pennsylvania

Howard K. Rabinowitz, James J. Diamond, Mohammadreza Hojat, and Christina E. Hazelwood

While prior studies have identified a number of factors individually related to physician practice in rural areas, little information is available regarding the relative importance of these factors or their relationship to rural retention. Extensive data previously collected from the Jefferson Longitudinal Study were analyzed for 1972–1992 graduates of Jefferson Medical College (JMC) practicing in Pennsylvania in 1996, as were recent self-reported perceptions of JMC graduates in rural practice. Rural background was overwhelmingly the most important independent predictor of rural practice, and freshman plan to enter family practice was the only other independent predictor. No other variable, including curriculum or debt, added significantly to the likelihood of rural practice. None of these variables, however, including rural background, were predictive of retention, which appeared to be more related to practice issues such as income and workload. The results suggest not only that increasing the number of physicians who grew up in rural areas is the most effective way to increase the number of rural physicians, but also that any policy that does not include this may be unsuccessful.

The Journal of Rural Health, 1999, *15*, 212–218. https://jdc.jefferson.edu/cgi/viewcontent.cgi?referer=&httpsredir=1&article=1068&context=hpn

1.2.11 Using Postgraduate Clinical Performance to Monitor Change in the Medical School

J. Jon Veloski

To study the impact of curricular changes and changes in admission policy upon the performance of Jefferson graduates, three stages of analysis were used to address each issue. The first stage was the multivariate analysis of variance comparing the appropriate groups simultaneously on four areas of competence, followed by one-way analysis of variance and post hoc tests.

To determine the effect of an increase in the number of female medical school graduates, data were analyzed on all women entering Jefferson between 1966 and 1973. This group of female students was compared with a random sample of men matched with the year of entry, type of premedical program, and ethnicity. Analysis of variance identified a difference between men and women only in the areas of professional attitudes. Twice as many female residents as male residents were rated in the top quarter on general effectiveness in dealing with people and nearly twice as many female residents were rated in the top quarter on being able to deal with patient and family tensions.

The accelerated premedical curriculum was examined to see whether or not there were deleterious effects resulting from a considerably shortened premedical education. The accelerated student group did not score as high as the control groups on general effectiveness in dealing with people or on the ability to handle patient/family tensions. The accelerated group did not rate in the top quarter on an item dealing with a sense of humor. Overall, the students entering medical school on an accelerated program showed no significant deficits in clinical effectiveness.

Proceedings of the Eighteenth Annual Conference on Research in Medical Education, Washington, DC. 1979, 425.
This abstract was written by the book editors.

1.2.12   Baccalaureate Preparation for Medical School: Does Type of Degree Make a Difference?

Carter Zeleznik, Mohammadreza Hojat, and J. Jon Veloski

Four groups of medical school matriculants (43 with a BA degree in social science, 68 with a BA degree in humanities, 49 with a BA degree in science, and 40 with a BS degree in science) were studied. No significant difference was found among the four groups on yearly grade-point averages in medical school or on Parts I, II, and III of the examinations of the National Board of Medical Examiners. Those with an undergraduate degree in the humanities considered leaving medical school more frequently than the others. A substantial proportion of medical students with an undergraduate major in the sciences and social sciences reported that they would choose humanities if they were once again high school seniors. Those with a science background were disproportionately more likely than the others to choose residencies in internal medicine and surgery, and those with undergraduate degrees in humanities and social sciences were more likely to choose psychiatry residencies.

Journal of Medical Education, 1983, *58*, 2633. https://pubmed.ncbi.nlm.nih. gov/6848754/#:~:text=No%20significant%20difference%20was%20 found,more%20frequently%20than%20the%20others

1.2.13   Levels of Recommendation for Students and Academic Performance in Medical School

Carter Zeleznik, Mohammadreza Hojat, and J. Jon Veloski

Traditionally, letters of recommendation from undergraduate institutions have been considered a major criterion for admission to medical school. Little attention, however, has been directed to the relationship between the content of their recommendation and measures of performance in medical school. This study was designed to determine whether or not such a relationship exists.

Letters of recommendation for 236 students who came to Jefferson from five different undergraduate institutions were reviewed and the level of recommendation contained in each letter was identified. These were compared with the yearly GPAs, scores on three parts of the National Board of Medical Examiners, and ratings of performance in the first year of residency training. Simple correlational, multiple regression, and factor analyses all indicated that the level of the recommendation did not contribute significantly to the ability to predict the medical student's academic performance.

Psychological Reports, 1983, *52*(3), 851–858.

Chapter 2
Demographics

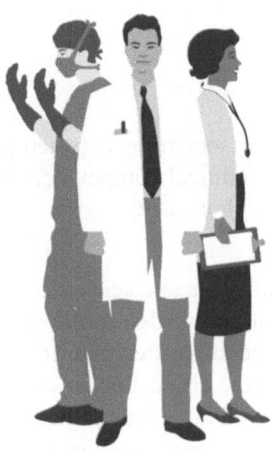

Contents

2.1 Standardized Patient Assessment of Medical Student Empathy: Ethnicity and
     Gender Effects in a Multi-institutional Study.. 30
2.2 Gender Segregation by Specialty During Medical School............................. 31
2.3 Comparing the Accuracies of Entire-Group and Subgroup Model to Predict NBME
     I Scores for Medical School Applicants.. 32
2.4 African-American and White Physicians: A Comparison of Satisfaction with
     Medical Education, Professional Careers, and Research Activities.................... 33
2.5 Performance and Career Expectations of Women Medical Students: A Comparison
     with Men.. 34
2.6 Gender Comparisons of Medical Students' Psychosocial Profiles...................... 35
2.7 Gender Comparisons of Income Expectations in the USA at the Beginning of
     Medical School During the Past 28 Years.. 36
2.8 Salary Inequities and Healthcare Costs.. 37
2.9 Gender Comparisons of Young Physicians' Perceptions of Their Medical
     Education, Professional Life, and Practice: A Follow-Up Study of Jefferson
     Medical College Graduates.. 38
2.10 Gender Comparisons Prior to, During, and After Medical School Using Two
     Decades of Longitudinal Data at Jefferson Medical College.......................... 39
2.11 Change of Interest in Surgery During Medical School: A Comparison of Men and
     Women.. 40
2.12 Prediction of Students' Performance on Licensing Examinations Using Age, Race,
     Sex, Undergraduate GPAs, and MCAT Scores.. 41
2.13 A National Study of Factors Influencing Primary Care Career Choices Among
     Underrepresented Minority, White, and Asian-American Physicians.................... 42
2.14 Performance on the NBME Part I Examination.. 43

2.15   Board Certification: Associations with Physicians' Demographics and
       Performances During Medical School and Residency................................... 44
2.16   Longitudinal Comparison of the Academic Performances of Asian-American
       and White Medical Students... 45

Abstract

This chapter describes findings on associations between gender, age, and race/ethnicity with academic performance, clinical competence, specialty interest, interaction with patient, and satisfaction with **career.**

Gender
- Men outscored women on quantitative and science tests prior to medical school, and on examinations of medical knowledge in the preclinical phase of medical school; however, no significant gender difference was observed in faculty assessments of clinical competence in the clinical phase of medical education.
- No gender difference was observed on attrition rates in medical school.
- Gender comparisons of personality profiles showed that women scored significantly higher than men on measures of general anxiety, test anxiety, and neuroticism, but lower on loneliness experiences.
- Women consistently outscored men in self-reported clinical empathy.
- Women appraised stressful life events more negatively than men.
- Men reported higher satisfaction than women in their decision to choose medicine.
- Compared to men, women assigned lower priority to economic values and financial incentive factors, but valued psychological aspects of patient care more than men.
- Women were more likely to work part-time, and less inclined to practice highly paid specialties. Female medical students expected lower annual peak income than men.

Age
- Students' age did not correlate significantly with performance measures.
- Certification rates were lower among older and underrepresented minority graduates.

Race/Ethnicity
- African-American graduates were comparable with their White counterparts on their reported satisfaction with medical education and medical career.
- Asian/Pacific Islander compared with White students had significantly higher mean scores on the Scholastic Aptitude Test (SAT), and science subtests of the MCAT, with the exception of MCAT reading subtest in which White students outscored their Asian/Pacific Islander counterparts. Asian/Pacific Islander students did not perform as well as White classmates on medical licensing examinations.

- No significant difference was observed between the Asian/Pacific Islander and White ethnic groups on ratings of clinical competence given by residency program directors in the first year of postgraduate training.
- Significant differences were observed among African-American, Asian/Pacific Islander, and White students on self-reported empathy in favor of the African-American group. However, male African-American students obtained the lowest ratings on empathy by standardized patients, regardless of standardized patients' race/ethnicity.

Keywords African-American · Age · Asian-American · Board certification · Career plan · Change of interest · Gender · Healthcare costs · Income expectation · National Board Medical Examiners' examinations · Primary care career choice · Professional life · Psychosocial profiles · Race/ethnicity · Salary inequalities · Satisfaction with medical school · Specialty interest · Standardized patient · Underrepresented minorities

2.1   Standardized Patient Assessment of Medical Student Empathy: Ethnicity and Gender Effects in a Multi-institutional Study

*Katherine Berg, Benjamin Blatt, Joseph Lopreiato, Julianna Jung,
Arielle Schaeffer, Daniel Heil, Tamara Owens, Pamela L. Carter-Nolan,
Dale Berg, J. Jon Veloski, Elizabeth Darby, and Mohammadreza Hojat*

Purpose: To examine, primarily, the effects of ethnicity and gender, which could introduce bias into scoring on standardized patient (SP) assessments of medical students and, secondarily, to examine medical students' self-reported empathy for ethnicity and gender effects so as to compare self-perception with the perceptions of SPs.

Method: Participants were 577 students from four medical schools in 2012: 373 (65%) were White, 79 (14%) Black/African American, and 125 (22%) Asian/ Pacific Islander. These students were assessed by 84 SPs: 62 (74%) were White and 22 (26%) were Black/African American. SPs completed the Jefferson Scale of Patient Perceptions of Physician Empathy (JSPPPE) and the Global Ratings of Empathy tool. Students completed the Jefferson Scale of Empathy and two Interpersonal Reactivity Index subscales. The investigators used 2882 student-SP encounters in their analyses.

Results: Analyses of SPs' assessments of students' empathy indicated significant interaction effects of gender and ethnicity. Female students, regardless of ethnicity, obtained significantly higher mean JSPPPE scores than men. Female Black/African-American, female White, and female Asian/Pacific Islander students scored significantly higher on the JSPPPE than their respective male counterparts. Male Black/African-American students obtained the lowest SP assessment scores of empathy regardless of SP ethnicity. Black/African-American students obtained the highest mean scores on self-reported empathy.

Conclusions: The significant interaction effects of ethnicity and gender on clinical encounters, plus the inconsistencies observed between SPs' assessments of students' empathy and students' self-reported empathy, raise questions about possible ethnicity and gender biases in the SPs' assessments of medical students' clinical skills.

Academic Medicine, 2015, *90*(1), 105–111. https://doi.org/10.1097/ ACM.0000000000000529

2.2   Gender Segregation by Specialty During Medical School

Ann Boulis, Jerry Jacobs, , and J. Jon Veloski

In this retrospective cohort study from the University of Pennsylvania, USA, the authors examined how gender segregation across specialties has changed during the past 20 years and how gender segregation changes during medical school. Data from the Jefferson Longitudinal Study of Medical Education on 4312 medical students' specialty choices before, during, and after medical school were analyzed. Women constituted 26.7% of students in the sample. Intended specialty choices were limited to (1) anesthesiology, pathology, and radiology, referred to as hospital-based specialties; (2) emergency medicine; (3) family practice; (4) internal medicine; (5) obstetrics-gynecology; (6) ophthalmology; (7) pediatrics; (8) psychiatry; (9) surgery; (10) other; and (11) undecided. There was a significant trend toward increased gender segregation among specialties between the 1980s and 1990s, with an increased concentration of men in surgery, hospital specialties, and internal medicine, and an increased concentration of women in pediatrics, family practice, and obstetrics-gynecology. Also, there was an increase in gender-based segregation during medical school that the authors attributed primarily to the large percentage of students (over one-third) who enter medical school without a specialty preference and who ultimately distribute themselves across specialties in a gender-segregated way. Seventy-nine percent of female students and 75% of male students were either undecided initially or changed specialties during medical school. The authors say that for the vast majority of students the medical school experience not only had the potential to influence their choice of specialty, but also played a role in the gender-based segregation of specialty choice among students.

Academic Medicine, 2001, 76(10), S65–S67. https://doi.org/10.1097/00001888-200110001-00022

2.3   Comparing the Accuracies of Entire-Group and Subgroup Model to Predict NBME I Scores for Medical School Applicants

James B. Erdmann, Mohammadreza Hojat, and J. Jon Veloski

To address the question of whether prediction models for subgroups of medical school applicants lead to more accurate predictions of performance than does one model for an entire group of applicants, the authors used data from two groups of students at Jefferson Medical College: 415 students who entered Jefferson in 1985 and 1986 and 396 who entered in 1987 and 1988. Both groups were divided into two subgroups by gender and two subgroups by age. Data from the first group were used to develop prediction models based on the entire group and on its four subgroups. The predictors were undergraduate grade-point averages and Medical College Admission Test scores; the criterion measures were scores on the National Board of Medical Examiners Part I examinations. The prediction models were then applied to data from the second group and its four subgroups; differences in the validity coefficients (0.40–0.56) and residual scores (7.2–17.9) were not considered to be of practical importance. Hence, the authors suggest that gender and age do not contribute to a prediction bias and that an entire-group prediction model can be used without serious concern for over- or underestimating the predicted scores.

Academic   Medicine,   1992,   *67,*   860–862.   https://doi.org/10.1097/
00001888-199212000-00014

2.4   African-American and White Physicians: A Comparison of Satisfaction with Medical Education, Professional Careers, and Research Activities

John Gartland, Mohammadreza Hojat, Edward B. Christian,
Clara A. Callahan, and Thomas J. Nasca

Background: Given the disparity between proportions of minority in the general population and in the physician workforce and the projected increase in the minority population, it is important and timely to examine factors that contribute to satisfaction of minority physicians.

Purpose: To examine similarities and differences between African-American and White physicians in their satisfaction with medical school, their medical careers, and their professional and research activities and achievements.

Methods: A questionnaire was mailed to the 148 active African-American graduates of Jefferson Medical College (1960–1995). Control group was 148 active White classmates matched as to gender, year of graduation, and scores on Step 2 of the United States Medical Licensing Examination (formerly Part II of the National Board).

Results: Overall response rate was 61% (African Americans 59%, White control group 63%). Both groups were equally satisfied with medical education, careers, and professional and research activities. No differences were noted between the groups in satisfaction with medical school financial support, preparation for a medical career, educational experience and academic environment, medical careers, and practice incomes. African Americans reported greater dissatisfaction than Whites with interactions with medical school faculty and administrators and with the medical school social environment. African Americans were less likely than Whites to recommend Jefferson to minority applicants and to contribute to Annual Alumni Giving. More African Americans than Whites practiced medicine in economically deprived areas and cared for poor minority patients.

Conclusions: African-American respondents were comparable with White respondents as to their medical careers, professional activities, and achievements as physicians. Their practice patterns reflected a greater sense of community need and involvement than their White counterparts. The sense of dissatisfaction with the social environment of medical school noted by African-American respondents seems to persist during their professional careers.

Teaching and Learning in Medicine, 2003, *15*(2), 106–112. https://www.tandfonline.com/doi/abs/10.1207/S15328015TLM1502_06

2.5 Performance and Career Expectations of Women Medical Students: A Comparison with Men

Mary W. Herman and J. Jon Veloski

In this study, data are presented pertaining to the performance and career expectations of women who entered medical school between 1966 and 1968. Women are compared with men, both as a point of reference for general trends and to measure changes in sex differences. The data were derived from an ongoing longitudinal study of medical students at Jefferson Medical College. No significant differences were found between the sexes in attrition or in measures of clinical competence. Significant differences between men and women in expected hours of work and years of professional activity disappear in the latter part of the study period. Women have lower income expectations, and more of them plan to work in small communities in the latter time period, but they do not differ from men in the proportions interested in primary care specialties or clinical careers. Both sexes showed, over time, increased interest in family medicine and working in small communities.

The New England Journal of Medicine (Letter to the Editor), 1980, *302*, 1035–1036.
   This abstract was written by the book editors.

2.6   Gender Comparisons of Medical Students' Psychosocial Profiles

Mohammadreza Hojat, Karen Glaser, Gang XuJ. Jon Veloski,
and Edward B. Christian

Objectives: This study was designed to compare male and female medical students on selected personality attributes that could influence their academic attainment and personal success.

Design: Participants were 1157 medical students (743 men, 414 women) who completed a set of psychosocial questionnaires measuring intensity and chronicity of loneliness, general anxiety, test anxiety, neuroticism, depression, extraversion, self-esteem, locus of control, perceptions of parents, general health, and appraisals of stressful life events. Data were analyzed by employing multivariate and univariate analysis of variance and chi-square analysis.

Setting: Jefferson Medical College

Subjects: Medical Students

Results: Men scored significantly higher on the intensity of loneliness, and women scored higher on general anxiety, test anxiety, and neuroticism scales, but the magnitudes of the effect size estimates were not large. No significant gender difference was observed on measures of chronicity of loneliness, depression, extraversion, self-esteem, external locus of control, and perception of the mother and the father. Women who experienced stressful life events, such as death in the family or personal illness, appraised these events more negatively than did their male counterparts.

Conclusions: Implications of the findings for medical education and practice are discussed.

Medical Education, 1999, *33*(5), 342–349. https://onlinelibrary.wiley.com/doi/full/10.1046/j.1365-2923.1999.00331.x

2.7   Gender Comparisons of Income Expectations in the USA at the Beginning of Medical School During the Past 28 Years

Mohammadreza Hojat, Joseph S. Gonnella, James B. Erdmann,
Susan L. Rattner, J. Jon Veloski, Karen Glaser, and Gang Xu

This study was designed to investigate gender differences in the USA in anticipated professional income. Participants were 5314 medical students (3880 men, 1434 women) who entered Jefferson Medical College between 1970 and 1997. The annual peak professional income estimated at the beginning of medical school was the dependent variable and gender within selected time periods was the independent variable. Results showed significant differences between men and women on their anticipated future incomes in different time periods. Women generally expected 23% less income than men. The effect size estimates of the differences were moderately high. The gender gap in income expectations was more pronounced for those who planned to pursue surgery than their counterparts who planned to practice family medicine or pediatrics. A unique feature of this study is that its outcomes could not be confounded by active factors such as experience, working hours, age, and productivity. Findings suggest that social learning may contribute to gender gap in anticipated income.

Social Science & Medicine, 2000, *50*(11), 1665–1672.
    Reprinted with permission from Elsevier.

2.8   Salary Inequities and Healthcare Costs

Mohammadreza Hojat, Joseph S. Gonnella, J. Jon Veloski, and Gang Xu

In response to a commentary on our findings from a follow-up study of our medi-cal school graduates to examine gender salary inequalities in physicians, we spec-ified the following points. Whether gender income gap is solely a function of socialization or other factors remains unclear. However, findings from the Jefferson Longitudinal Study suggest that there might be some endogenous in addition to exogenous factors that lead to gender income inequalities. For exam-ple, our findings indicated that women in medical school generally assigned a lower priority to economic values and financial incentive factors, and that female medical students anticipate a significantly lower peak professional income than their male counterparts. Furthermore, women physicians are more likely to work part-time, and on average work 40% fewer hours than men in their lifetimes, and are also less inclined to practice highly paid specialties. Although these findings may suggest that increasing number of women in medicine could contribute to decreased costs of health care, even if physicians' services constitute only a small portion of total healthcare expenditures, we neither endorse gender salary inequal-ities, nor recommend policies to maintain the trend. Indeed, we wholeheartedly recommend efforts to reduce the income gap between male and female physi-cians, and encourage further research to explore the intrinsic and extrinsic factors to narrow and eliminate the income gap.

Academic Medicine (Letter to the Editor), 1995, *70*(10), 853–854.
This abstract was written by the book editors.

2.9 Gender Comparisons of Young Physicians' Perceptions of Their Medical Education, Professional Life, and Practice: A Follow-Up Study of Jefferson Medical College Graduates

Mohammadreza Hojat, Joseph S. Gonnella, and Gang Xu

Purpose: To obtain information from a group of young physicians and compare men and women on their evaluations of selected areas of the medical school curriculum, their perceptions of issues related to medical practice and professional life, and their specialty choices, professional activities, and research productivity.

Method: In 1992, a questionnaire was mailed to 1076 physicians who had graduated from Jefferson Medical College between 1982 and 1986. The responses of men and women were compared using multivariate and univariate analyses of variance, t-tests, chi-square, and median test.

Results: Completed questionnaires were returned by 667 graduates (530 men and 137 women). The curriculum areas of interpersonal skills, disease prevention, medical ethics, and economics of health care were rated by both men and women as being the most important in medical training. Conversely, research methodology and statistics received the lowest ratings. Women, in general, valued psychosocial aspects of medical care higher than did men. Among the areas of perceived problems related to practice, lack of leisure time received the highest ratings (as being the greatest problem) and interpersonal interactions received the lowest ratings (as being the least problem) from both men and women. Men were more concerned than women about the areas of patient chart and documentation, malpractice litigation, physician oversupply, peer review, and interaction with patients. These differences remained when specialties and numbers of hours worked per week were held constant. Generally, the physicians reported satisfaction with their professional lives, but men tended to be more satisfied than women about their decisions to become physicians and in their perceptions of medicine as a rewarding career. The proportion of men employed full-time (99.4%) was significantly higher than that of women (84%). Women were more likely to practice general pediatrics, while men were more likely to practice surgery and surgical subspecialties. Full-time employed women worked fewer hours per week (57) than men (63), and men reported more research productivity than women.

Conclusion: The implications of the findings of numerous gender differences are discussed regarding the issues of physician workforce, types of care rendered by men and women, and possible changes in the national healthcare system.

Academic Medicine, 1995, *70*, 305–312. https://doi.org/10.1097/00001888-199504000-00014

2.10   Gender Comparisons Prior to, During, and After Medical School Using Two Decades of Longitudinal Data at Jefferson Medical College

Mohammadreza Hojat, Mary R. Robeson, J. Jon Veloski, Robert S. Blacklow, Gang Xu, and Joseph S. Gonnella

Similarities and differences prior to, during, and after medical school between 3541 male and 1121 female graduates of Jefferson Medical College were investigated. Gender comparisons were made on examination scores, admission interview ratings, competence ratings in residency, specialty choice, board certification, income estimates, and academic appointments. Results indicated that prior to medical school, women scored higher on verbal tests, whereas men outscored women on quantitative and science tests. During medical school, men performed better than women in the basic science examinations, but not in the clinical science examinations. Men and women had similar postgraduate competence ratings, except that women were rated higher than men in the socioeconomic aspects of patient care. Women had lower board certification rates, expected less income, and had a higher proportion of faculty appointments than men. Gender differences in specialty choices, faculty appointments, and estimated income could have important implications for healthcare manpower.

Evaluation & The Health Professions, 1994, *17*, 290–306.

2.11 Change of Interest in Surgery During Medical School: A Comparison of Men and Women

Karen Novielli, Mohammadreza Hojat, Pauline K. Park, Joseph S. Gonnella, and J. Jon Veloski

Problem statement and background: Women are underrepresented in the field of surgery. Reasons for this are incompletely understood.

Methods: Male and female graduates from a single medical school over the past three decades ($n = 4676$) were grouped by their interest in a surgical career at the beginning and the end of medical school. Factors associated with choice of a surgical residency were compared.

Results: Compared to men, women were less likely to enter medical school interested in surgery, more likely to lose interest, and less likely to gain interest in surgery. Ratings of clinical competence in surgery clerkship were among the factors associated with losing or gaining interest in surgery. Income expectation was associated with gender and with a surgical career choice.

Conclusions: Retention and recruitment of medical students to surgery are significantly lower for women.

Academic Medicine, 2001, *76*(October Supplement), S58–S61. https://doi. org/10.1097/00001888-200110001-00020

2.12   Prediction of Students' Performance on Licensing Examinations Using Age, Race, Sex, Undergraduate GPAs, and MCAT Scores

J. Jon Veloski, Clara A. Callahan, Gang Xu, Mohammadreza Hojat, and David B. Nash

Purpose: To evaluate students' age, race, sex, undergraduate grades, and MCAT scores as predictors of licensing examination scores.

Method: Data for 30 classes ($n = 6239$) matriculating at a medical school between 1968 and 1997 were analyzed using multiple linear regression to predict NBME Parts I, II, and III and USMLE Steps 1, 2, and 3.

Results: The regression weight for MCAT science was 2–3 times that of MCAT verbal in predicting the first, preclinical examination. However, the weights for MCAT science, MCAT verbal, and science GPA were equal for the clinical and postgraduate tests. There was a negative weight associated with women on Part I, but positive weights on Steps 2 and 3. Being older showed no relationships. Every model yielded a negative weight for Asian-American students.

Academic Medicine, 2000, *75*(October Supplement), S28–S30. https://journals. lww.com/academicmedicine/Fulltext/2000/10001/Prediction_of_Students_ Performances_on_Licensing.9.aspx

2.13   A National Study of Factors Influencing Primary Care Career Choices Among Underrepresented Minority, White, and Asian-American Physicians

Gang Xu, Mohammadreza Hojat, J. Jon Veloski, and Jack Brose

This study examined the differences between three groups of physicians—underrepresented minority (URM), White, and Asian American—on factors that influenced their choice of primary care specialties. The groups were also compared with regard to their family backgrounds, financial aid obligations, educational debt, current practice settings, and level of satisfaction with their career choice. The general hypothesis was that, as URMs were more likely than Whites and Asians to grow up in underserved areas and to receive financial aid from the government for their medical education, their decision to choose primary care careers would be more influenced by their family background, receipt of financial aid, and obligations to serve in underserved areas. Clinical experiences with underserved patients may also have differentiated effects on different groups of physicians regarding their choice of primary care career.

Academic   Medicine,   1996,   *71*,   S10–S12.   https://doi.org/10.1097/
00001888-199610000-00029

2.14 Performance on the NBME Part I Examination

Gang Xu, J. Jon Veloski, and Mohammadreza Hojat

We examined data from the Jefferson Longitudinal Study by tracking academic and clinical performance of 12 classes of medical school in a commentary on a published study in which the question of why Asian/Pacific Islander medical students do not perform as well as White students on written tests such as Part I of the NBME was addressed. Our findings from this as well as another publication from the Jefferson Longitudinal Study showed that Asian/Pacific Islander medical students, compared to their White counterparts, had significantly higher mean scores in each of the MCAT subtests with the exception of the MCAT reading subtest. Also, Asian/Pacific Islander students performed lower than the White students not only in the NBME Part I, but also in Parts II and III. However, we found no statistically significant difference between Asian/Pacific Islander and their White counterparts on ratings of clinical competence given by the residency program director during the first year of residency training. In additional analyses using multiple regression, we found that the MCAT reading subtest score was the best predictor of the NBME Part I for Asian/Pacific Islanders; however, the MCAT science problems subtest score was the best predictor of the NBME Part I for the White medical students. Similar pattern of findings was also observed for predicting NBME Part II scores. We suggested that for better understanding of Asian/Pacific Islander medical students' performances on written examinations more attention should be given to measures of reading ability as possibly a confounding variable.

Journal of the American Medical Association (Letter to the Editor), 1995, *273*(8), 617–618.
This abstract was written by the book editors.

2.15   Board Certification: Associations with Physicians' Demographics and Performances During Medical School and Residency

Gang Xu, J. Jon Veloski, and Mohammadreza Hojat

Purpose: To examine the associations between board certification and both physicians' demographics and their performances during medical school and residency.

Method: Data were prospectively collected for 1186 medical students in three major specialty areas for the Jefferson Medical College's graduating classes of 1976 through 1985.

Results: Older students and underrepresented minorities were less likely to achieve certification. Overall, physicians who achieved board certification had performed better during medical school and residency than those without certification. The prediction of board certification using academic performance indicators is limited, particularly for older and minority groups.

Conclusions: This study demonstrated an overall positive relationship between physicians' board certification status and their past academic performances. The potential impact of the increase of both older students and minority physicians on rates of board certification needs to be considered by specialty boards and other policymakers.

Academic   Medicine,   1998,   *73*,   1283–1289.   https://doi.org/10.1097/00001888-199812000-00019

2.16   Longitudinal Comparison of the Academic Performances of Asian-American and White Medical Students

Gang Xu, J. Jon Veloski, Mohammadreza Hojat, Joseph S. Gonnella,
and Benjamin Bacharach

The purpose of the study was to compare the academic performances of Asian-American medical students—before, during, and after medical school—with those of White students. A total of 140 Asian-American graduates and 2269 White graduates from the classes of 1981–1992 at Jefferson Medical College were studied prospectively: data on academic performance, indebtedness, and delayed graduation were analyzed and compared for all the graduates. *F*-tests, chi-square tests, and regression models were used. The Asian Americans had statistically significantly higher scores on the Scholastic Aptitude Test (SAT) quantitative subtest and on the Medical College Admission Test (MCAT) chemistry, physics, and science problems subtests; the Whites had significantly higher scores on the MCAT reading subtest, third-year grade-point averages for required clerkships, and scores on the National Board of Medical Examiners Part I, II, and III examinations (NBME I, II, and III). No significant difference was found in the other performance measures, including ratings in the first year of residency. Regression analysis showed that the MCAT reading score was the major predictor of Asian Americans' performances on the NBME I and II.

Because the MCAT reading score is the major predictor of later performance for Asian-American students, schools should consider employing different criteria in predicting and monitoring these students' performances.

Academic Medicine, 1993, *68*, 82–86. https://pubmed.ncbi.nlm.nih.gov/8447898/
Reprinted (in Chinese) in *International Medicine*, 1993, *4*, 179–183.

Chapter 3
Medical School Evaluations

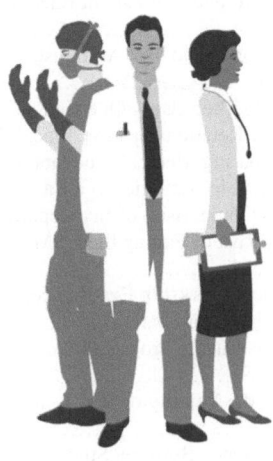

Contents

3.1   Preclinical.. 50
    3.1.1   An Empirical Study of the Predictive Validity of Number Grades in Medical
        School Using Three Decades of Longitudinal Data: Implications
        for a Grading System.. 50
    3.1.2   The Fate of Medical Students with Different Levels of Knowledge: Are
        the Basic Medical Sciences Relevant to Physician Competence?............... 51
    3.1.3   Sooner or Later? USMLE Step 1 Performance and Test Administration Date
        at the End of the Second Year.. 52
    3.1.4   Using Ratings of Resident Competence to Evaluate NBME Examination
        Passing Standards.. 53
3.2   Clinical... 54
    3.2.1   Students' Ratings of Otolaryngology Clerkship Activities: The Role
        of Residents... 54
    3.2.2   A Comparison of Medical Students' Self-Reported Empathy
        with Simulated Patients' Assessments of the Students' Empathy................ 55
    3.2.3   The Relationship Between Performance on a Medical School's Clinical
        Skills Assessment and USMLE Step 2 CS... 56
    3.2.4   Validity of Faculty Ratings of Students' Clinical Competence in Core
        Clerkships in Relation to Scores on Licensing Examinations
        and Supervisors' Ratings in Residency... 57
    3.2.5   Subtest Scores of a Comprehensive Examination of Medical Knowledge
        as a Function of Retention Interval... 58

3.2.6   Evaluation of the Validity of Medical Students' Self-Assessments
         of Proficiency in Clinical Simulations... 59
3.2.7   Students' Gender and Examination of Patients in a Third-Year Family
         Medicine Clerkship.. 60
3.2.8   Evaluations of Medical Students' Clinical Experiences in a Family
         Medicine Clerkship: Differences in Patient Encounters by Disease Severity
         in Different Clerkship Sites... 61
3.2.9   USMLE Step 2 Performance and Test Administration Date in the Fourth
         Year of Medical School.. 62
3.2.10   A Comparison of the Modified Essay Question and Multiple-Choice
         Question Formats: Their Relationships to Clinical Performance.................. 63
3.2.11   Documenting and Comparing Medical Students' Clinical Experiences.......... 64
3.2.12   Student Ratings of Clerkship Activities as a Basis for Curriculum
         Modification: A 4-Year Comparison of Six Departments......................... 65
3.2.13   Identifying Students at Risk of Failing the USMLE Step 2 Clinical Skills
         Examination... 66
3.2.14   Evaluation of the Surgical Clerkship Experience in Affiliated Hospitals:
         Performance on Objective Examinations... 67
3.2.15   Do Global Rating Forms Enable Program Directors to Assess the ACGME
         Competencies?.. 68
3.2.16   A Preliminary Study of the Validity of Scores and Pass/Fail Standards
         for USMLE Steps 1 and 2... 69
3.2.17   Evaluation of the Congruence Between Students' Postencounter Notes
         and Standardized Patients' Checklists in a Clinical Skills Examination.......... 70
3.2.18   Attendings' and Residents' Teaching Role and Students' Overall Rating
         of Clinical Clerkships... 71
3.2.19   Influence of Previous Clerkship Experiences on Students' Satisfaction
         with Their Current Clerkship.. 72
3.2.20   A Correlation Study of Students' Perception of Their Active Role
         as Related to Their Clerkship Experiences... 73

Abstract

- Studies of the psychometric properties of the routine assessments of students conducted throughout the curriculum have been the underpinning of the study. This research included published investigations of clinical competence and the factors linked to it—formal knowledge examinations, performance in clinical simulations, and faculty ratings of student performance under supervision in clinical settings.
- Multiple published studies examined the validity of scores on examinations early in students' medical education as predictors of their scores on national licensing examinations.
- Studies of the association between examination scores early in medical education concluded that low scores were important indicators of subsequent low performance ratings by faculty members in clinical clerkships. These reinforced the relevance of the basic medical sciences to the formation of clinical competence.

- Reported also are systematic studies of these young physicians' performance in residency training soon after leaving medical school. Correspondingly, these provided evidence of the effectiveness of the curriculum and the validity of the assessments developed by faculty throughout the curriculum.
- Several methodological studies focused on the congruence between faculty assessments of students in clerkships and comprehensive assessments of their competence using clinical simulations with standardized patients at completion of their core clerkships. These indicated that the clinical simulations measured abilities that were different from the proficiency of students in clerkships.
- On the other hand, there were studies of the quality and rigor of clinical clerkships as reflected in the students' ratings of their clinical experiences and detailed reports of patient encounters.
- Studies initiated in the 1970s provided empirical evidence that students could achieve the objectives of the curriculum though clinical rotations in diverse patient care settings ranging from the university hospital to local affiliated hospitals and remote community hospitals.
- Numerous studies were led by faculty members involved in the curriculum, but based outside of the center, to foster faculty development. These addressed issues such as students' risk of failing licensure examinations based on records of their Jefferson grades and timely academic progress through the curriculum.
- A study of the widely assumed validity of students' self-assessments of their performance in clinical simulations revealed that the weakest students were more likely to overestimate the standardized patients' ratings of their clinical competence.

Keywords Clinical competence · Core clerkships · Delayed graduation · Dismissal · Documentation of clinical experiences · Empathy · Faculty ratings · Failure rate · Grading systems · Medical licensing examinations · Modified essay examinations · Numerical versus letter grades · Knowledge acquisition examination · Objective Structured Clinical Examination (OSCE) · Overall satisfaction · Pass-fail grades · Patient encounter · Performance assessments · Physician competence · Predictive validity · Residency supervisor ratings · Retention · Simulated patient · Standardized patient · United States Medical Licensing Examination (USMLE)

3.1   Preclinical

3.1.1   An Empirical Study of the Predictive Validity of Number Grades in Medical School Using Three Decades of Longitudinal Data: Implications for a Grading System

Joseph S. Gonnella, James B. Erdmann, and Mohammadreza Hojat

Context: It is important to establish the predictive validity of medical school grades. The strength of predictive validity and the ability to identify at-risk students in medical schools depend upon assessment systems such as number grades, pass/fail (P/F), or honors/pass/fail (H/P/F) systems.

Objective: This study was designed to examine the predictive validity of number grades in medical school, and to determine whether any important information is lost in a shift from number to P/F and H/P/F grading systems.

Subjects: The participants in this prospective, longitudinal study were 6656 medical students who studied at Jefferson Medical College over three decades. They were grouped into 10 deciles based on their number grades in year 1 of medical school.

Methods: Participants were compared on academic accomplishments in years 2 and 3 of medical school, medical school class rank, delayed graduation and attrition, performance on medical licensing examinations, and clinical competence ratings in the first postgraduate year.

Results: Results supported the short- and long-term predictive validity of the number grades. Ratings of clinical competence beyond medical school were predicted by number grades in medical school. We demonstrated that small differences in number grades are statistically meaningful, and that important information for identifying students in need of remedial education is lost when students who narrowly meet faculty's expectations are included with the rest of the class in a broad "pass" category.

Conclusions: The findings refute the argument that knowledge of sciences basic to medicine is not critical to subsequent performance in medical school and beyond if an appropriate evaluation system is used. Furthermore, the results of this study raise questions about abandoning number grades in favor of a pass/fail system. Consideration of these findings in policy decisions regarding assessment system of medical students is recommended.

Medical Education, 2004, *38*(4), 425–434. https://onlinelibrary.wiley.com/doi/10.1111/j.1365-2923.2004.01774.x

3.1.2 The Fate of Medical Students with Different Levels of Knowledge: Are the Basic Medical Sciences Relevant to Physician Competence?

Mohammadreza Hojat, Joseph S. Gonnella, James B. Erdmann, and J. Jon Veloski

Purpose: This study was designed to test the hypothesis that an early gap in knowledge of sciences basic to medicine could have a sustained negative effect throughout medical school and beyond.

Method: A longitudinal prospective study of 4437 students who entered Jefferson Medical College between 1972 and 1991 was conducted in which the students were divided into three groups. Group 1 consisted of 392 who failed at least one of the three basic sciences courses in the first year of medical school. Group II comprised of 398 who did not fail but had low first-year grade-point averages, and 3647 of the remaining sample were included in Group III. The groups were compared on retention and dismissal rates, medical school assessment measures, scores on medical licensing examinations, ratings of clinical competency in residency, board certification rates, and faculty appointments.

Results: Significant differences were observed among the three groups confirming the hypothesis that students' level knowledge in sciences basic to medicine early in medical school could predict later performance during medical school and beyond. Implications for early diagnosis of academic deficiencies, for better preparation of medical students, and for assessment of clinical competency are discussed.

Advances in Health Sciences Education, 1996, *1*, 179–196. https://link.springer.com/article/10.1007/BF00162915

3.1.3   Sooner or Later? USMLE Step 1 Performance and Test Administration Date at the End of the Second Year

Charles A. Pohl, Mary R. Robeson, Mohammadreza Hojat, Susan L. Rattner, and J. Jon Veloski

Purpose: To determine whether the elapsed time between completion of the second-year curriculum and test date alters a student's outcome on USMLE Step 1.

Methods: Total scores for 601 students who completed Step 1 in 1999–2001 were classified into six, 1-week time periods between June 1 and mid-July depending on the test date. Analysis of variance and covariance was used to explore differences across time with adjustment for previous academic performance.

Results: Mean weekly scores decreased from a high of 221 in early June to a low of 208 in July. However, analysis of covariance confirmed that differences across time were not significant ($p < 0.30$). Weekly differences were explained by predicted performance based on gender, MCAT science, and medical school test scores.

Conclusions: Performance on Step 1 is unaffected by the time interval between completing the curriculum and taking the examination within the first 2 months after completing the preclinical curriculum.

Academic Medicine, 2002, 77, S17–S19.
https://journals.lww.com/academicmedicine/Fulltext/2002/10001/Sooner_or_Later__USMLE_Step_1_Performance_and_Test.6.aspx

3.1.4 Using Ratings of Resident Competence to Evaluate NBME Examination Passing Standards

Barbara J. Turner, Mohammadreza Hojat, and Joseph S. Gonnella

The passing standards of the NBME examinations were empirically evaluated by analyzing the distribution of scores received by 1994 graduates of one medical school and the clinical competence ratings given to the graduates by their first-year residency directors. A significant association was found between NBME scores and postgraduate ratings in the cognitive areas of clinical competence. Graduates scoring 420 or less on NBME Part I or II received significantly lower medical knowledge ratings than did the total group of graduates. A similar analysis of NBME Part III scores was less clear-cut but also suggested that a score of 420 or less could identify those graduates at significant risk of receiving lower knowledge ratings. Using low cognitive ratings as an outcome measure, NBME Part II was not sensitive in detecting such graduates. Based on these data, changes in passing standards could not be proposed, but rather the authors recommended that these standards continue to be reassessed and further measures be taken to strengthen the internal evaluation methods in medical schools.

Journal of Medical Education, 1987, *62*(7), 572–581. https://doi.org/10.1097/00001888-198707000-00006

3.2   Clinical

3.2.1   Students' Ratings of Otolaryngology Clerkship Activities: The Role of Residents

Hidemichi Ashikawa, Gang Xu, and J. Jon Veloski

This study was conducted with a sample of junior medical students at Jefferson Medical College to investigate the factors that influence students' overall satisfaction with the otolaryngology clerkship. The most important factor related to their overall satisfaction in the clerkship was their experience with residents, followed by experience with attending physicians, quality of rounds, and lectures. The number of patients the students encountered and the number of rounds and lectures were deemed less important. Based on these findings, the authors of this paper concluded that the residents' role in teaching should be emphasized and students' satisfaction with the otolaryngology clerkship may be enhanced by developing residents' skills in teaching students.

Medical   Teacher,   1992,   *14*,   77–81.   https://www.tandfonline.com/doi/abs/10.3109/01421599209044019

3.2.2 A Comparison of Medical Students' Self-Reported Empathy with Simulated Patients' Assessments of the Students' Empathy

Katherine Berg, Joseph F. Majdan, Dale Berg, Jon Veloski,
and Mohammadreza Hojat

Background: Empathy is necessary for communication between patients and physicians to achieve optimal clinical outcomes.

Aim: To examine associations between simulated patients' (SPs) assessment of medical students' empathy and students' self-reported empathy.

Methods: A total of 248 third-year medical students completed the Jefferson Scale of Physician Empathy (JSPE). SPs completed the Jefferson Scale of Patient Perceptions of Physician Empathy (JSPPPE), and a global rating of empathy in 10 objective clinical skills examination encounters during a comprehensive end of third-year clinical skills examination.

Results: High correlation was found between the scores on the JSPPPE and the global ratings of empathy completed by the SPs ($r = 0.87$, $p < 0.01$). A moderate but statistically significant correlation was observed between scores of the JSPE and the JSPPPE ($r = 0.19$, $p < 0.05$). Significant differences were observed on the JSPE and global ratings of empathy among top, middle, and low scorers on the JSPPPE in the expected direction.

Conclusions: While significant associations exist between students' self-reported scores on the JSPE and SPs' evaluations of students' empathy, the associations are not large enough to conclude that the two evaluations are redundant.

Medical Teacher, 2011, *33*(5), 388–391. https://www.tandfonline.com/doi/full/10.3109/0142159X.2010.530319

3.2.3   The Relationship Between Performance on a Medical School's Clinical Skills Assessment and USMLE Step 2 CS

Katherine Berg, Marci Winward, Brian E. Clauser, Judith A. Veloski, Dale Berg, Gerald F. Dillon, and J. Jon Veloski

Background: Little is known about the relationship between performance on clinical assessments during medical school and performance on similar licensing tests.

Method: Correlation coefficients were computed and corrected for measurement error using data for 217 students who completed a school's clinical assessment and took the Step 2 clinical skills (CS) examination.

Results: Observed (and corrected) correlations between the two tests were 0.18 (0.32) for data gathering, 0.35 (0.75) for documentation, and 0.32 (0.56) for communication/interpersonal skills. The highest correlation within each test was between documentation and data gathering. The lowest was between documentation and communication/interpersonal skills.

Conclusions: The pattern of correlations supports each test's construct validity. The low correlations suggest that the tests are not redundant, and do not support using the scores on the school's assessment to predict performance on Step 2 CS. Future studies of these relationships need to address the time between the two assessments and the effect of intervening remedial programs.

Academic Medicine, 2008, *83*(10), S37–S40. https://doi.org/10.1097/ACM.0b013e318183cb5c

3.2.4 Validity of Faculty Ratings of Students' Clinical Competence in Core Clerkships in Relation to Scores on Licensing Examinations and Supervisors' Ratings in Residency

Clara A. Callahan, James B. Erdmann, Mohammadreza Hojat, J. Jon Veloski, Susan L. Rattner, Thomas J. Nasca, and Joseph S. Gonnella

Problem Statement and Background: The validity of the clinical evaluations in medical school, a major component of the dean's letter, as an independent predictor of postgraduate clinical competence, has not been well documented.

Method: In a cohort study, 2156 medical students at Jefferson Medical College who graduated from 1989 to 1998 were studied. Bivariate and multivariate relationships between competence ratings in third-year core clerkships, performance on licensing examinations, and residency program directors' ratings of clinical competence were examined.

Results: Significant correlations were found between clerkship ratings and criterion measures. Clerkship ratings in internal medicine, family medicine, pediatrics, and obstetrics/gynecology yielded higher correlations than psychiatry and surgery.

Conclusions: These results should not only increase the confidence of the faculty about their evaluations, but also assure residency selection committees about the validity of such evaluations in predicting clinical competence beyond medical school.

Academic Medicine, 2000, *75*(October Supplement), S71–S73. https://journals.lww.com/academicmedicine/Fulltext/2000/10001/Validity_of_Faculty_Ratings_of_Students__Clinical.23.aspx

3.2.5   Subtest Scores of a Comprehensive Examination of Medical Knowledge as a Function of Retention Interval

Mohammadreza Hojat and J. Jon Veloski

It was hypothesized that performance on particular subtests of a comprehensive examination would be a function of the length of time between the completion of medical training and administration of the comprehensive examination. Two samples of graduates of the Jefferson Medical College were studied: one group of 1086 students who graduated between 1975 and 1979, and another group of 877 who graduated between 1980 and 1983. Each medical student in the junior year was assigned to one of four clerkship groups. Each group took the assigned clerkship training in internal medicine, obstetrics/gynecology, pediatrics, psychiatry, and surgery in a different rotational sequence. Statistical analyses indicated that there were no significant differences among the four groups of the two samples on total comprehensive medical examination scores either before or after the junior year. There was, however, a linear trend found in the scores on subtests in psychiatry, obstetrics/gynecology, and surgery in both samples. The trend indicated that the shorter the interval between clerkship training and the examination, the higher the score on that particular examination. Data were analyzed in terms of some hypotheses from learning theories, and the implications of the results on medical education were discussed.

Psychological Reports, 1984, *55*, 579–585.

Copyright© 1984. Sage Publishing. https://journals.sagepub.com/doi/10.2466/pr0.1984.55.2.579?icid=int.sj-abstract.similar-articles.3

Also in *Proceedings of the Twenty-Second Annual Conference on Research in Medical Education*, Washington, DC. November 1983, 19–24.

3.2.6   Evaluation of the Validity of Medical Students' Self-Assessments of Proficiency in Clinical Simulations

Gerald A. Isenberg, Vibin Roy, J. Jon Veloski, Katherine Berg, and Charles J. Yeo

Background: The accuracy of self-assessments has not been well supported in the literature. This study was undertaken to examine the validity of medical students' ratings of their proficiency during encounters with simulated patients and simulation devices.

Methods: Confidential self-assessments for 10 skills were collected from 195 students during a formal clinical skills assessment related to 3 cases at the end of a surgery clerkship. The cases required students to gather data from simulated patients and perform procedures such as rectal examinations, nasogastric tube insertions, and suturing on bench simulation models. The patients were trained to assess student performance.

Results: There were significant differences between student self-assessments and simulated patient scores for general clinical skills as opposed to procedural skills. Students' mean self-assessments in the data gathering and interpersonal skills were 2–6% points higher than ratings of their proficiency by simulated patients. However, self-assessments on procedures were 5–8 points lower than patient ratings. The median correlation between self-assessments and patient ratings for general clinical skills such as data gathering and interpersonal skills was 0.08 (not significant), whereas the median correlation between student and patient ratings in procedures was 0.22 ($p < 0.01$).

Conclusions: Third-year medical students' self-assessments for specific procedures are more valid than self-assessments of general clinical skills. Students are less confident in their procedural skills compared with general clinical skills. Although self-assessments should not be used as the sole measure of performance in clinical simulations, self-assessments for specific procedures can provide supplemental information on proficiency.

Journal of Surgical Research, 2015, *193*(2), 554–559. https://www.journalofsurgicalresearch.com/article/S0022-4804(14)00894-4/fulltext

3.2.7 Students' Gender and Examination of Patients in a Third-Year Family Medicine Clerkship

Daniel Z. Louis, Jonathan Gottlieb, Fred W. Markham, Mohammadreza Hojat, Carol Rabinowitz, and Joseph S. Gonnella

The present study investigated gender differences in clinical experiences measured by the number of times a specific set of diagnostic, therapeutic, and preventive tasks was performed as part of a required clerkship in medical school. Participants were 194 third-year medical students at Jefferson Medical College who were taking their required 6-week family medicine clerkship during the 1994–1995 academic year. There were 117 men (60%) and 77 women (40%) in this group. We used specially designed computer-scannable patient-encounter cards to document students' clinical experiences. The patient-encounter cards were designed as part of a broad study to monitor students' clinical experiences in required clerkships and to ensure that all students are sufficiently exposed to diverse clinical situations and perform the diagnostic, therapeutic, and preventive tasks relevant to each clerkship. A total of 16,570 patient encounters (60% female patients) were reported by 194 students. A total of 9425 patient-encounter cards were completed by male students. A total of 7185 patient-encounter cards were completed by female students. There was no difference between male and female students with respect to the proportion of male and female patients encountered, but female students encountered significantly more patients overall than male students. The mean number of patient encounters reported per student was 85 (81 for male students, 93 for female students) over a 6-week period. A significantly larger percentage of women than men (91% vs. 65%) performed at least one breast examination in their family medicine clerkship ($p < 0.01$). However, men were more likely than women to perform a testicular examination (71% of the men and 58% of the women, $p < 0.05$). Women also performed the Denver Developmental Screening Test for children more often than men (58% of the women and 43% of the men, $p < 0.05$). Women were more likely than men to perform pelvic examinations (84% of the women vs. 73% of the men, $p < 0.10$), but the difference fell short of statistical significance at the conventional level. The results of this study show that while men and women in a family medicine clerkship are exposed to a patient base with comparable gender composition, certain diagnostic tasks are not performed as often by male and female students.

Academic   Medicine,   1996,   *71*(Supplement),   S19–S21.   https://doi. org/10.1097/00001888-199610000-00032

3.2.8   Evaluations of Medical Students' Clinical Experiences in a Family Medicine Clerkship: Differences in Patient Encounters by Disease Severity in Different Clerkship Sites

Fred W. Markham, Susan L. Rattner, Mohammadreza Hojat, Daniel Z. Louis, Carol Rabinowitz, and Joseph S. Gonnella

Background and Objectives: Evaluation of medical students' clinical encounters is an essential component of optimizing their educational experience. In this study, we collected data on the diagnoses and disease severity in student-patient encounters at different family medicine clerkship sites.

Methods: Participants were 582 third-year medical students who completed a total of 7515 specially designed patient-encounter cards in a 6-week family medicine clerkship at five training sites over 3 years.

Results: Variation was found in the average number of encounters in different clerkship sites. The findings for three frequently encountered diseases (essential hypertension, diabetes mellitus, and upper respiratory infection) showed significant differences in the proportions of patients at different stages of the disease in different clerkship sites.

Conclusions: Students at different clerkship sites experience different numbers of encounters with patients and significant variation in the illness severity of patients seen in those encounters.

Family Medicine, 2002, *34*(6), 451–454.

3.2.9   USMLE Step 2 Performance and Test Administration Date in the Fourth Year of Medical School

Charles A. Pohl, Mary R. Robeson, and J. Jon Veloski

Purpose: To determine whether the time interval between completing the third-year curriculum and test administration affects a student's USMLE Step 2 score.

Method: Scores for 846 students in the classes of 2000–2004 were grouped in 10 time periods depending on test date. A linear regression model to predict performance on Step 2 using gender, Step 1, and grades in medicine, pediatrics, and obstetrics-gynecology was developed based on the class of 1999. Analysis of covariance was used to test the effect of time on scores, adjusting for predicted performance.

Results: Step 2 scores decreased significantly ($p < 0.001$) across time. Students' mean scores were four points higher than predicted in the early months and five to eight points lower near the end of the senior year.

Conclusions: Students who scheduled Step 2 early in the senior year achieved higher scores, on average, than those who waited until later in the year.

Academic Medicine, 2004, *79*(10), S49–S51. https://doi.org/10.1097/0000 1888-200410001-00015

3.2.10 A Comparison of the Modified Essay Question and Multiple-Choice Question Formats: Their Relationships to Clinical Performance

Howard K. Rabinowitz and Mohammadreza Hojat

The Department of Family Medicine at Jefferson Medical College has been using the modified essay question as the final examination format for its required third-year clerkship since 1976. To compare the family medicine modified essay question format with the multiple-choice question format used in the other five required junior clerkships, examination scores from 2174 Jefferson graduates (1976–1985) were correlated with scores on the examination of the National Board of Medical Examiners (NBME), ratings of clinical performance in the required third-year clerkships, and ratings on four global areas of postgraduate competence. Grades of the multiple-choice examination in internal medicine consistently yielded the highest correlations with NBME scores and with postgraduate ratings of medical knowledge. Performance on the modified essay examination in family medicine had the lowest correlations in these areas. The family medicine scores, however, consistently yielded the highest correlations with overall third-year clinical performance and with postgraduate performance in the areas of data gathering skills, clinical judgment, and professional attitudes. These results indicate that the modified essay question format may provide a different and important parameter in the evaluation of medical trainees.

Family Medicine, 1989, *21*, 364–367.

3.2.11   Documenting and Comparing Medical Students' Clinical Experiences

Susan L. Rattner, Daniel Z. Louis, Carol Rabinowitz, Jonathan E. Gottlieb,
Thomas J. Nasca, Fred W. Markham, Ruth P. Gottlieb, John W. Caruso,
J. Lindsey Lane, J. Jon Veloski, Mohammadreza Hojat , and Joseph S. Gonnella

Context: The decentralization of clinical teaching networks over the past decade calls for a systematic way to record the case mix of patients, the severity of diseases, and the diagnostic procedures that medical students encounter in clinical clerkships.

Objective: To demonstrate a system that documents medical students' clinical experiences across clerkships.

Design and Settings: Evaluation of a method for recording student-patient clinical encounters using a pocket-sized computer-read patient-encounter card at a US university hospital and its 16 teaching affiliates during academic years 1997–1998 through 1999–2000.

Participants: A total of 647 third-year medical students who completed patient-encounter cards in three clerkships: family medicine, pediatrics, and internal medicine.

Main Outcome Measures: Number of patient encounters, principal and secondary diagnoses, severity of diseases, and diagnostic procedures as recorded on patient-encounter cards; concordance of patient-encounter card data with medical records.

Results: Students completed 86,011 patient-encounter cards: 48,367 cards by 582 students in family medicine, 22,604 cards by 469 students in pediatrics, and 15,040 cards by 531 students in internal medicine. Significant differences were found in students' case mix of patients, level of disease severity, and number of diagnostic procedures performed across the three clerkships. Stability of findings within each clerkship across 3 academic years and 77% concordance of students' reports of principal diagnosis with faculty's confirmation of diagnosis support the reliability and validity of the findings.

Conclusions: An instrument that facilitates students' documentation of clinical experiences can provide data on important differences among students' clerkship experiences. Data from this instrument can be used to assess the nature of students' clinical education.

Reprinted with permission from *Journal of the American Medical Association*, 2001, *286*(9), 1035–1040.

3.2.12   Student Ratings of Clerkship Activities as a Basis for Curriculum Modification: A 4-Year Comparison of Six Departments

Joseph S. Rodgers, J. Jon Veloski, and Shelley L. Moses

This study was undertaken to determine which activities and learning experiences have the greatest positive influence on students' overall ratings of the educational values of clinical clerkships. Such results could provide guidance to curriculum committees, faculty of individual departments, and those responsible for clinical education in hospitals who must set priorities and plan changes in clerkships.

The self-reports of students expressed on 3634 forms collected over a 4-year period provide an opportunity to investigate the relative importance of different learning experiences in required clinical clerkships. Most significant across the clerkships is the learning value placed on patient rounds. In five of the six clerkships, students who gave high overall ratings to the clerkship also reported frequently that patient rounds were valuable. Such data do support the learning value of rounds and probably also the concept that student learning is enhanced when the entire time of rounds is devoted to teaching medical students. On the other hand, certain variables did not appear to influence students' overall rating of the clerkship experience. The value of conferences, whether or not a student was given time off to study prior to the final examination, the number of hours on call, and the number of new patients per week showed little or no relationship to the students' overall ratings of clerkships. The results also suggest that more emphasis should be placed on the role of the attending physician. The program should be so constructed as to enable attending physicians to spend more time with students, especially discussing their assigned patients. Feedback to students, which they have perceived as important but lacking in other studies, should be included.

Proceedings of the Twenty-Sixth Annual Conference on Research in Medical Education, Washington, DC. November 1987, 179–184.
This abstract was written by the book editors.

3.2.13 *Identifying Students at Risk of Failing the USMLE Step 2 Clinical Skills Examination*

Susan Rosenthal, Stefani Russo, Katherine Berg, Joseph Majdan, Jennifer Wilson, Charlotte Grinberg, and J. Jon Veloski

Background and Objectives: New standards announced in 2017 could increase the failure rate for Step 2 clinical skills (CS). The purpose of this study was to identify student performance metrics associated with the risk of failing.

Methods: Data for 1041 graduates of one medical school from 2014 through 2017 were analyzed, including 30 (2.9%) failures. Metrics included Medical College Admission Test, the United States Medical Licensing Examination Step 1, and clerkship National Board of Medical Examiners (NBME) subject examination scores; faculty ratings in six clerkships; and scores on an Objective Structured Clinical Examination (OSCE). Bivariate statistics and regression were used to estimate the risk of failing.

Results: Those failing had lower Step 1 scores, NBME scores, faculty ratings, and OSCE scores ($p < 0.02$). Students with four or more low ratings were more likely to fail compared to those with fewer low ratings (relative risk [RR], 12.76, $p < 0.0001$). Logistic regression revealed other risks: low surgery NBME scores (RR 3.75, $p = 0.02$), low pediatrics NBME scores (RR 3.67, $p = 0.02$), low ratings in internal medicine (RR 3.42, $p = 0.004$), and low OSCE communication/interpersonal skills (RR 2.55, $p = 0.02$).

Conclusions: Certain medical student performance metrics are associated with the risk of failing Step 2 CS. It is important to clarify these and advise students accordingly.

Family Medicine, 2019, *51*(6), 483–499.

3.2.14 Evaluation of the Surgical Clerkship Experience in Affiliated Hospitals: Performance on Objective Examinations

Gordon F. Schwartz, J. Jon Veloski, and Joseph S. Gonnella

This study was designed to measure the knowledge acquired during the surgical clerkship required in the third-year curriculum at Jefferson Medical College and to determine whether or not that knowledge varied according to the institution in which it was acquired. Student grades were derived from scores of 0–100 in each of the four subtests: surgery, orthopedics, urology, and anesthesiology. Grades were grouped by hospital, and means and variances were computed for each institution. Significant differences for the entire group of hospitals were observed in three of the subtests. It can be inferred that, based on the apparent differences in knowledge among students assigned to several hospitals, differences may occur in clinical competence and attitudes.

Journal of Surgical Research, 1976, *20*, 179–182.
Reprinted with permission from Elsevier.

3.2.15   Do Global Rating Forms Enable Program Directors to Assess the ACGME Competencies?

*Cynthia G. Silber, Thomas J. Nasca, David L. Paskin, Glenn Eiger,
Mary R. Robeson, and J. Jon Veloski*

Purpose: In 1999 the Accreditation Council for Graduate Medical Education (ACGME) mandated that GME programs require their residents to be proficient in six general competencies. The purpose of this study was to ascertain whether an existing global rating form could be modified to assess these competencies.

Method: A rating form covering 23 skills described in the ACGME competencies was developed. The directors of 92 specialty and subspecialty programs at Thomas Jefferson University Hospital and the Albert Einstein Medical Center in Philadelphia were asked to rate residents at the end of the 2001–2002 and 2002–2003 academic years.

Results: Ratings for 1295 of 1367 (95%) residents were available. Residents were awarded the highest mean ratings on items tied to professionalism, compassion, and empathy. The lowest mean ratings were assigned for items related to consideration of costs in care and management of resources. Factor analysis indicated that the program directors viewed overall competence in two dimensions of medical knowledge and interpersonal skills. This factor structure was stable for groups of specialties and residents' gender and training level. Mean ratings in each dimension were progressively higher for residents at advanced levels of training.

Conclusion: Global rating forms, the tool that program directors use most frequently to document residents' competence, may not be adequate to assess the six general competencies. The results are consistent with earlier published research indicating that physicians view competence in just two broad dimensions, which questions the premise of the six ACGME competencies. Further research is needed to validate and measure six distinct dimensions of clinical competence.

Academic Medicine, 2004, 79(6), 549–556.   https://doi.org/10.1097/0000
1888-200406000-00010

3.2.16   A Preliminary Study of the Validity of Scores and Pass/ Fail Standards for USMLE Steps 1 and 2

David B. Swanson, Susan M. Case, Donna Waechter, J. Jon Veloski,
Carol Hasbrouck, Miriam Friedman, Jan Carline, and Carol Maclaren

Medical licensure in the USA is in a period of transition. In 1991, the National Board of Medical Examiners (NBME) introduced major modifications in the content, format, pass/fail standards, and score reports for the NBME Part I and Part II examinations. In 1992, the modified Part I and Part II examinations were renamed Step 1 and Step 2 and became the first two components of the three-step United States Medical Licensing Examination (USMLE). When the Part Examinations and the Federation Licensing Examination (FLEX), developed by the Federation of State Medical Boards (FSMB), completely phased out in 1994, the USMLE became the sole examination pathway to initial licensure for allopathic physicians.

As a part of the phase-in of the revised examinations in 1991, new pass/fail standards for Part I and Part II were instituted. These standards were predominantly content based: the score required to pass was determined primarily by reviewing test items and identifying a level of performance reflecting mastery of the materials. In 1992, these new standards were adopted for administrations of USMLE Steps 1 and 2. The purpose of this project was to initiate systematic study of the correspondence between performance on the examinations and academic achievement in basic science coursework and clinical clerkships during medical school. In this preliminary study, examinees' scores and pass/fail results from the first administrations of the newly designed Part I and Part II were compared with ratings of academic achievement provided by five collaborating medical schools.

Academic   Medicine,   1993,   *68*,   S19–S21.   https://doi.org/10.1097/0000
1888-199310000-00033

3.2.17   Evaluation of the Congruence Between Students' Postencounter Notes and Standardized Patients' Checklists in a Clinical Skills Examination

Katherine Worzala, Susan L. Rattner, John R. Boulet, Joseph F. Majdan, Dale D. Berg, Mary Robeson, and J. Jon Veloski

Background and Purpose: Questions remain about the congruence between students' written notes and checklists as summaries of encounters.

Methods: Students examined standardized patients and summarized findings in postencounter notes. The patients completed checklists. A physician read the students' notes and completed parallel checklists to document the history and physical items performed. Rates of under- and overdocumentation were calculated.

Results: Students documented findings for 71% of items performed—an underdocumentation rate of 29%. Approximately 94% of their documented findings were consistent with what they had done. Their rate of overdocumentation was 6%, in which they documented findings inconsistent with the checklists. About half the students had no instances of overdocumentation.

Conclusion: Students' rate of underdocumentation was comparable to experienced clinicians. Although their overdocumentation rate was low overall, it was high for a few students. Evaluation of the congruence between checklists and postencounter notes provides useful information and informs checklist development.

Teaching and Learning in Medicine, 2008, *20*(1), 31–36. https://www.tandfonline.com/doi/full/10.1080/10401330701798253

3.2.18 Attendings' and Residents' Teaching Role and Students' Overall Rating of Clinical Clerkships

Gang Xu, Timothy P. Brigham, J. Jon Veloski, and Joseph F. Rodgers

The study was conducted with a sample of third-year students ($n = 584$) at Jefferson Medical College to explore students' perception of patterns of differences between attending physicians and residents in their teaching behaviors during clinical clerkships. Attending physicians' teaching behaviors were perceived more in a mentorship mode whereas residents' teaching behaviors were equally divided between mentorship and preceptorship modes. Attending physicians' and residents' teaching behaviors varied among clerkships. Results were discussed in terms of difference of teaching roles played by attending physicians and residents and relationship of the teaching behaviors to students' overall rating of clerkship.

Medical Teacher, 1993, *15*, 217–222.
https://www.tandfonline.com/doi/abs/10.3109/01421599309006716?journalCode=imte20

3.2.19   Influence of Previous Clerkship Experiences on Students' Satisfaction with Their Current Clerkship

Gang Xu and J. Jon Veloski

This study examined the influence of previous clerkship experiences on students' satisfaction with their current clerkship. We hypothesized that when students are asked to rate their current clerkship, their ratings are influenced by their comparisons of current experiences with previous ones, whether or not they are asked to make such comparisons.

We surveyed the 225 third-year students at our school at the end of the last block in 1991–1992. The students were asked to give (1) their overall ratings of the clerkship; (2) their ratings of experiences in 19 activities, such as experiences with attending physicians, with residents, on rounds, in conferences, etc.; and (3) their ratings of the clerkship in comparison with previous clerkships.

Experiences in previous clerkships influence students' satisfaction with their experiences in subsequent clerkships.

Medical educators, in order to gain a better understanding of their students' experiences in the clerkships of their own departments, should look into the students' experiences in the clerkships of other departments.

Academic Medicine, 1993, *68*, 230. https://journals.lww.com/academicmedicine/Abstract/1993/03000/Influence_of_previous_clerkship_experiences_on.18.aspx

3.2.20   A Correlation Study of Students' Perception of Their Active Role as Related to Their Clerkship Experiences

Gang Xu, J. Jon Veloski, and Timothy P. Brigham

Previous studies have indicated the importance of students' active involvement in clinical learning. This study examined medical students' active participation in clinical clerkships as related to their ratings of clerkship experiences. The general hypothesis is that students' perception of being active in the clerkship will be positively related to their experience with attendings and residents and to their overall satisfaction with their clerkship experience. This hypothesis was examined in teaching rounds, work rounds, and in conferences and was confirmed in the study. Future study may be needed to explore specific approaches to bring students into an active process in different clinical learning settings.

Medical Teacher, 1995, *17*, 199–203.   https://www.tandfonline.com/doi/abs/ 10.3109/01421599509008308

Chapter 4
Postgraduate and Career

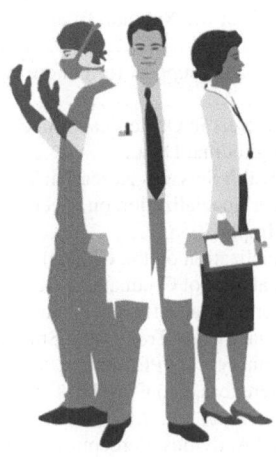

Contents

4.1   Clinical Competence.. 79
    4.1.1   Class Ranking Models for Deans' Letters and Their Psychometric Evaluation... 79
    4.1.2   Further Psychometric Evaluations of a Class Ranking Model as a Predictor
        of Graduates' Clinical Competence in the First Year of Residency............... 80
    4.1.3   Relationship Between Performance in Medical School and Postgraduate
        Competence.. 81
    4.1.4   A Case of Mistaken Identity: Signal and Noise in Connecting Performance
        Assessments Before and After Graduation from Medical School................. 82
    4.1.5   What Have We Learned and Where Do We Go from Here?....................... 83
    4.1.6   Assessment Measures in Medical School, Residency, and Practice:
        The Connections... 84
    4.1.7   The Role of Resident Performance Evaluation in Board Certification............ 85
    4.1.8   Measuring the Contribution of Medical Education to Patient Care: A Review.... 86
    4.1.9   Validity and Importance of Low Ratings Given to Medical School Graduates
        in Noncognitive Areas... 87
    4.1.10 Cognitive and Noncognitive Factors in Predicting the Clinical Performance
        of Medical School Graduates... 88
    4.1.11 Is the Glass Half Full or Half Empty? A Reexamination of the Associations
        Between Assessment Measures During Medical School and Clinical
        Competence After Graduation.. 89
    4.1.12 Components of Postgraduate Competence: Analyses of 30 Years
        of Longitudinal Data... 90
    4.1.13 Components of Clinical Competence Ratings of Physicians: An Empirical
        Approach.. 91

4.1.14   Conceptualization and Measurement of Clinical Competence of Residents:
         A Brief Rating Form and Its Psychometric Properties.   92
4.1.15   Relationships Between Performance in Medical School and First
         Postgraduate Year.   93
4.1.16   Affirmative Action and Special Consideration Admissions to Medical
         Education.   94
4.1.17   A Validity Study of Part III of the National Board Examination.   95
4.2   Specialization and Professional Activities.   96
4.2.1   Correlates of Young Physicians' Support for Unionization to Maintain
         Professional Influence.   96
4.2.2   Stability and Change of Interest in Obstetrics-Gynecology Among Medical
         Students: 18 Years of Longitudinal Data.   97
4.2.3   Medical Education and Health Services Research: The Linkage.   98
4.2.4   The Impact of Early Career Specialization on Licensing Requirements
         and Related Educational Implications.   99
4.2.5   The Impact of Early Specialization on the Clinical Competence of Residents. . .   100
4.2.6   Should Half of All Medical School Graduates Enter Primary Care?
         Perceptions of Faculty Members at Jefferson Medical College.   101
4.2.7   Family Medicine and Primary Care: Trends and Student Characteristics.   102
4.2.8   Primary Care and Non-primary Care Physicians: A Longitudinal Study
         of Their Similarities, Differences, and Correlates Before, During, and After
         Medical School.   103
4.2.9   Differences in Professional Activities, Perceptions of Professional Problems,
         and Practice Patterns Between Men and Women Graduates of Jefferson
         Medical College.   104
4.2.10   A Program to Increase the Number of Family Physicians in Rural
         and Underserved Areas: Impact After 22 Years.   105
4.2.11   Critical Factors for Designing Programs to Increase the Supply
         and Retention of Rural Primary Care Physicians.   106
4.2.12   Who Is a Generalist? An Analysis of Whether Physicians Trained
         as Generalists Practice as Generalists.   107
4.2.13   A Statewide System to Track Medical Students' Careers: The Pennsylvania
         Model.   108
4.2.14   Generalist Career Plans: Tracking Medical School Seniors Through
         Residency.   109
4.2.15   Choice of First-Year Residency Position and Long-Term Generalist Career
         Choices.   110
4.2.16   Assessment of Physicians' Interest in Primary Care Training/Retraining.   111
4.2.17   Changing Specialties: Do Anesthesiologists Differ from Other Physicians?. . .   112
4.2.18   Migration of Physicians to and from Anesthesiology.   113
4.2.19   Academic Performance of Psychiatrists Compared to Other Specialists
         Before, During, and After Medical School.   114
4.2.20   Board Certification in Obstetrics and Gynecology: Associations
         with Physicians' Demographics and Performances During Medical School. . .   115
4.2.21   Performance on the NBME Part II Examination and Career Choice.   116
4.2.22   Medical Students Who Enter General Surgery Residency Programs:
         A Follow-Up Between 1972 and 1986.   117
4.2.23   Perceptions of Practice Problems Encountered by Family Physicians,
         Pediatricians, and Orthopedic Surgeons.   118
4.2.24   Primary Care and Non-primary Care Physicians' Concerns in Practice
         and Perceptions of Medical School Curriculum.   119
4.2.25   Factors Associated with Changing Levels of Interest in Primary Care
         During Medical School.   120

4.2.26 Emergency Medicine Career Change: Associations with Performances
        in Medical School and in the First Postgraduate Year and with Indebtedness.. 121
4.2.27 The Changing Healthcare System: A Research Agenda for Medical
        Education.. 122
4.2.28 A National Study of the Factors Influencing Men and Women Physicians'
        Choices of Primary Care Specialties.. 123
4.2.29 A Comparison of Jefferson Medical College Graduates Who Chose
        Emergency Medicine with Those Who Chose Other Specialties................ 124
4.2.30 Factors Influencing Physicians' Decisions to Remain in Emergency
        Medicine.. 125
4.2.31 Comparing the Academic Performances of Geriatricians and Other Family
        Physicians and Internists.. 126
4.2.32 Comparisons Among Three Types of Generalist Physicians: Personal
        Characteristics, Medical School Experiences, Financial Aid, and Other
        Factors Influencing Career Choice.. 127
4.2.33 Changing Interest in Family Medicine and Students' Academic Performance. 128
4.2.34 Physicians' Intention to Stay in or Leave Primary Care Specialties
        and Variables Associated with Such Intention.................................. 129
4.2.35 Factors Influencing Primary Care Physicians' Choice to Practice
        in Medically Underserved Areas... 130
4.2.36 Factors Influencing Physicians' Choices to Practice in Inner-City or Rural
        Areas.. 131

Abstract

- The investigators in these published follow-up studies made innovative use of the Longitudinal Study's vast database on the residency education, specialization, sub-specialization, and professional careers of Jefferson graduates over more than five decades. In particular, this unique resource includes comprehensive data on all Jefferson graduates since 1968 from the AMA's Physician Master File of self-reported career activities and the certification and recertification records of the ABMS.

- Using program directors' ratings of the graduates during their first year of residency, several studies were designed to validate the methods used to compile medical students' class rank and support their applications for residency programs.

- Several studies investigated graduates' changes in specialization, trends in graduates' interest in particular specialties, and personal characteristics and academic credentials of graduates who entered the new specialties of family medicine and emergency medicine after they were created in the 1970s.

- Long-term follow-up studies of Jefferson graduates in rural practice settings produced substantial empirical evidence that attracted a broad national readership. The findings supported the efficacy of Jefferson's innovative, long-standing Physician Shortage Area Program that systematically admitted applicants with a commitment to practice in rural communities. At Jefferson, these students pursued elective clerkships in rural settings and were subsequently more likely to provide care to patients in rural areas.

- Another long-term follow-up was designed to identify the early risk factors associated with physicians' unprofessional conduct. This case-control study included data from two other medical schools. Although low in prevalence, the physicians who were cited for unprofessional conduct by their state licensing boards decades after graduation were more likely to have been observed by Jefferson faculty to have a low capacity for self-improvement.

Keywords Affirmative action · Board certification · Career choice · Class ranking · Components of competence · Early specialization · Emergency medicine · Family medicine career · Gender comparisons · Generalist career · Health services research · Inner city and rural areas · Measures of clinical skills · Medical education and patient care · Noncognitive measures · Performance assessment · Personality measures · Physician competence · Physician shortage area program · Physician unionization · Postgraduate competence · Preferential admission · Primary care · Psychosocial measures · Specialty interest · Underserved areas

4.1   Clinical Competence

4.1.1   Class Ranking Models for Deans' Letters and Their Psychometric Evaluation

Robert S. Blacklow, Carla E. Goepp, and Mohammadreza Hojat

The dean's letter of evaluation written on behalf of graduating medical students is considered an important document in evaluating applicants to postgraduate residency programs. A recurrent complaint of those who must interpret deans' letters is that too often it is impossible to estimate how a candidate performed in comparison with his or her peers. One approach to providing such comparative information is to report the class rank in the body of the letter.

Despite the importance of comparative performance information, no serious attention has been directed toward developing a model to incorporate performance data in basic science as well as clinical science components of medical education in determining the class rank and to relate this to actual performance as a resident. The purpose of this study was to develop class ranking models in which performance data from both basic and clinical sciences could be used and to analyze the predictive validity of the models.

The total study sample consisted of 1283 graduates from Jefferson Medical College between 1986 and 1991. Five models were developed in determining the class rank. Different weights for basic and clinical science performance measures were employed in each model. Performance data from the first and second years (basic science component of medical education) and the third year (clinical sciences) were utilized in each model. Average ratings on each of the three areas of postgraduate competence—data gathering and processing skills, interpersonal skills, and socioeconomic aspects of patient care—were used as criterion measures for the validity study.

Validity of the models was studied by examining the true-positive and true-negative rates based on the distribution of ranking models and ratings on the postgraduate competence areas. In this approach, for each ranking model, the top 25% and bottom 25% of the graduates were chosen. Also, the top and bottom 25% of the graduates, based on the distribution of each postgraduate competence area, were chosen. A model in which a weight of one-third was assigned to basic science grades and a weight of two-thirds to the clinical ratings in medical school showed more satisfactory true-positive and true-negative rates. This model represented a more acceptable balance between weights assigned to performance measures in basic and clinical sciences.

Academic Medicine, 1991, *66*(Supplement), S10–S12. https://journals.lww.com/academicmedicine/Citation/1991/09001/Class_Ranking_Models_for_Deans_Letters_and_Their.5.aspx

Also in *Proceedings of the Thirtieth Annual Conference on Research in Medical Education*, Washington, DC. November 1991.

4.1.2   Further Psychometric Evaluations of a Class Ranking Model as a Predictor of Graduates' Clinical Competence in the First Year of Residency

Robert S. Blacklow, Carla E. Goepp, and Mohammadreza Hojat

This study was designed to investigate further the psychometrics of a class ranking model in which a weight of one-third was assigned to performance measures in basic sciences and a weight of two-thirds to ratings on six core clerkships. The first part of the study involved 215 graduates of Jefferson Medical College who, based on the ranking model, had been in the top and bottom quarters of the classes of 1991 and 1992. Six faculty, who did not know the graduates' ranks but were familiar with their performances and characteristics, were asked to judge the graduates' potentials to become competent physicians. The graduates' ranks according to the model were then compared with the ratings they received from the faculty. The second part of the study investigated whether there was a linear relationship between class ranks and ratings of postgraduate competence, by using directors' ratings of the data gathering skills of 598 graduates (1986–1990) at the end of their first year of residency. A concordance rate of 85% was obtained between the graduates' ranks and the ratings they received from the medical school faculty, which supports the criterion-related validity of the ranking model. In addition, class ranks were linearly related to ratings of postgraduate competence. However, women and graduates who had been low achievers in medical school were less likely to have given permission for collecting postgraduate ratings, which led to range restriction and a possible underestimation of the validity of the model. The psychometric evidence supports the class ranking model, but other schools should exercise caution in employing the model until they accumulate evidence from data obtained from their own students.

Academic Medicine, 1993, *68*, 295–297.   https://doi.org/10.1097/00001888-199304000-00017

4.1.3   Relationship Between Performance in Medical School and Postgraduate Competence

Joseph S. Gonnella and Mohammadreza Hojat

A sample of 441 graduates (between 1971 and 1981) of Jefferson Medical College who pursued their medical training in internal medicine, pediatrics, and obstetrics/ gynecology was selected. It was hypothesized that the relationship between measures of academic achievement in medical school and measures of postgraduate performance would vary in different specialty programs. The hypothesis was confirmed by comparing graduates in the three specialties on grades in medical school, scores on the examinations of the National Board of Medical Examiners, and ratings in four areas of competence in the first postgraduate year (that is, medical knowledge, data gathering skills, clinical judgment, and professional attitudes). It was also hypothesized that the strength of the relationship would vary at different levels of performance within the specialty programs. This was confirmed for some of the variables. The results indicated that inappropriate conclusions may be drawn about the relationship between performance before and after graduation from medical school if specialty differences and levels of performance are ignored.

Journal of Medical Education, 1983, *58*, 679–685. https://psycnet.apa.org/record/ 1984-15992-001

4.1.4 A Case of Mistaken Identity: Signal and Noise in Connecting Performance Assessments Before and After Graduation from Medical School

Joseph S. Gonnella, Mohammadreza Hojat, James B. Erdmann, and J. Jon Veloski

The authors examine the assumption that there is continuity from one level of training to another in structured and purposeful professional education. Thus, more advanced levels of training are built upon the foundations laid in the preceding levels. While the connection between performance before and performance after graduation from medical school is theoretically rational, such a connection has not been well documented in empirical studies. The issue has been debated but has not been settled because relevant findings are inconsistent. It is argued that these inconsistencies can stem from contaminating factors and the conceptual and methodological limitations of empirical studies. Such limitations are described in terms of "noise" that obscures the maximal value of a true relationship (the "signal"). Contaminating factors such as the time interval between testing; institutional factors; specialty choices; conceptual dissimilarities between performance measures in medical school and in practice; methodological limitations such as the shapes of rating distributions, nonlinearity, heteroscedasticity, restriction of range, multicollinearity, voluntary participation, psychometrics of assessment instruments, and differing methods of assessments; and a lack of assessments of personal qualities can produce "noise" that inhibits the strength of the "signal." While suggesting solutions for extricating some of the tangled web of methodological and conceptual issues, the authors feel that solutions do not exist for all of the problems. They conclude that researchers should be aware of the limitations if they are to avoid underestimating the "signal," which may fade because of background "noise."

Academic Medicine, 1993, *68*(Supplement), S9–S16. https://doi.org/10.1097/00001888-199302000-00023

4.1.5 What Have We Learned and Where Do We Go from Here?

Joseph S. Gonnella, Mohammadreza Hojat, James B. Erdmann, and J. Jon Veloski

Longitudinal data from five medical schools—Jefferson Medical College, Medical College of Georgia, Southern Illinois University, University of Missouri at Kansas City, and Wright State University—were combined in a meta-analytic study to investigate the global associations between performance measures in medical schools and clinical competence in residency. The total number of physicians from the five schools was 858, and top and bottom scorers in medical schools were divided into top and bottom groups based on their clinical competence ratings given by the directors of residency programs. It was found that 75% of high achievers in medical school were also rated high in clinical competence in their first year of residency. Of the low achievers in medical school, 61% were also rated low in their residency. The sensitivity and specificity of the combined data from the five medical schools were 0.74 and 0.63, respectively. An effect size of 0.36 was obtained. The results supported the proposition that associations between assessment measure during medical school and ratings of clinical competence in residency exist to a significant degree. Important factors in determining physician's competence were discussed and suggestions were made for future studies concerning performance measures in medical school and their connections to clinical competence beyond medical school.

Academic Medicine, 1993, *68*(Supplement), S79–S87. https://doi.org/10.1097/00001888-199302000-00036
  Also in Gonnella, J.S., Hojat, M., Erdmann, J.B., & Veloski, J.J. (1993). (Eds.). *Assessment measures in medical school, residency and practice: The connections.* (Chapter 15, pp. 155–173) New York: Springer.

4.1.6   Assessment Measures in Medical School, Residency, and Practice: The Connections

Joseph S. Gonnella, Mohammadreza Hojat, James B. Erdmann, and J. Jon Veloski

This collection of articles on the relationships between assessment measures in medical school, residency training, and practice of medicine was first published as a thematic special issue of *Academic Medicine*, and subsequently was reprinted as an independent book by Springer. The Jefferson team served as invited editors of this monogram that specifically addressed the issue of the relationships between performance in medical school, residency training, and practice of medicine. This theme was a logical extension of a long debate among medical educators over the relevance of medical education to the practice of medicine. In response to a call for papers and invitations to those whose ideas were more relevant to the theme, the editors received a large number of proposals. In the final volume, a group of 29 national and international medical education researchers shared their thoughts or contributed empirical research using data from their own academic medical centers. The volume contains three articles on nonempirical perspectives, and ten empirical studies.

Data from the Jefferson Longitudinal Study were used in a key article, using a large sample of 2368 graduates of the Jefferson Medical College (now Sidney Kimmel Medical College), confirming significant associations between measures of performance in medical school (e.g., basic science courses in the first- and second-year, clinical science examinations in the third-year, and ratings of clinical competence in the third-year core clerkships) and ratings of clinical competence, given by the residency program directors at the completion of the first residency year (using the Jefferson postgraduate rating form). Authors of four other studies from other medical schools also reported a similar pattern of findings of significant associations between measure of performance during and after medical school, summarized in the Epilogue section of the volume. Benefitting from our experiences and empirical evidence from the Jefferson Longitudinal Study, this is a unique document in medical education research that provides evidence from five medical schools using similar research methodology to show significant associations between performance measures in medical school and beyond. The findings, thereby, increase the confidence of medical school faculty that their assessments have predictive validity beyond medical school.

Assessment Measures in Medical School, Residency, and Practice: The Connections. New York: Springer Publishing Company, 1993.

Originally published as a special supplement in *Academic Medicine*, 1993, *68*(February Supplement).

4.1.7 The Role of Resident Performance Evaluation in Board Certification

Joseph S. Gonnella, Mohammadreza Hojat, James B. Erdmann, and J. Jon Veloski

The essence of graduate medical education involves mentoring, which implies continuous evaluation of a resident's performance accompanied by constructive feedback to enhance its development. The process should begin early in the program with a diagnostic assessment of the relevant competencies followed up by an educational plan leading to the desired outcome. The fact that residents and fellows are committed to 3 or more years of graduate medical education in the same organization presents a unique opportunity for program leaders to evaluate performance systematically. The number of years that residents spend in the same program, unlike the weeks that medical students spend rotating among multiple departments, enables more thorough evaluation of residents together with remedial work when necessary.

Evaluation criteria for resident performance must be clearly defined and embraced by the specialty boards and the programs to support formative and summative evaluations. A competent physician fills a triad of roles. An acceptable evaluation must assess the resident's performance in each of the three capacities: clinician, patient education, and manager of resources. Not only is it essential that each resident leave the program with the required clinical skills, but it is also important that the resident be able to communicate effectively with patients to clarify their medical programs, develop a management plan devised to improve their health, and achieve the expected outcomes of their care, including any risks. Lately, it has become even more important that the resident also acquire business and managerial skills to use resources efficiently and to understand the economic constraints facing medicine. A model for specifying the competencies of clinician, patient educator, and resource manager is proposed.

Certain factors that affect healthcare outcomes but fall outside of the physician's direct control also need to be understood and considered when evaluating performance. These include the contributions of other members of the healthcare team, availability of technology in different settings, capacity of the patient and family to collaborate in the care plan, and constraints imposed by insurance coverage or government regulation. A thorough and accurate evaluation of a resident's performance must take these factors into account.

From a methodical perspective, some tightening of the rationale for determining acceptable performance standards is also recommended. Most programs and boards have defensible standards for deciding if a specific competency has been achieved. What may be questioned, however, are evaluation schemes that permit above-average performance in one essential competency to offset less than adequate performance in another essential area, with the result that overall performance is judged acceptable.

Mancall, E.L. and Bashook, P.G. (1998). (Eds.), *Evaluating Residents for Board Certification* (pp. 3–14). Chicago, IL: American Board of Medical Specialties.
This abstract was written by the book editors.

4.1.8   Measuring the Contribution of Medical Education
to Patient Care: A Review

Joseph S. Gonnella, Mohammadreza Hojat, J. Jon Veloski, and Carter Zeleznik

This invited review describes the specific contribution that medical education makes to patient care. Although most studies conducted over the past 30 years have reported that the link between the education of physicians and their professional competence is negligible, limitations in those analyses require investigation. More recent empirical evidence from studies in which the Jefferson longitudinal database was used has indicated that a positive link exists between the levels at which medical students perform and the levels of competence at which they perform as physicians. This link is most evident when observations of the competence levels are made shortly after completing medical school. The reviewers found that many factors affect the ability to demonstrate the relationship between education and professional performance and these factors must be considered when research is undertaken.

Proceedings of the Twenty-second Annual Conference on Research in Medical Education, Washington, DC. November 1983, 3–16.
    This abstract was written by the book editors.

4.1.9 Validity and Importance of Low Ratings Given to Medical School Graduates in Noncognitive Areas

Mary W. Herman, J. Jon Veloski, and Mohammadreza Hojat

This study showed that the clinical ratings of noncognitive aspects of professional competence are generally valid. The ratings of 672 residents who graduated from Jefferson between 1978 and 1981, representing 76% of all graduates in that period, were analyzed. The ratings were made by chiefs of service, directors of medical education, or physicians who had the opportunity to closely observe the graduates in their residency setting. The study comprised ratings from 203 hospitals in the United States. Ten items on the rating form were identified as noncognitive, i.e., items dealing with attitudes and the ability to apply acquired knowledge. Overall, only 3% of the residents received low ratings on these items, and 40% of those received high ratings on at least two items. The validity of the ratings is tested by relating them to the willingness of residency supervisors to offer further postgraduate training to the graduate being evaluated and to the clinical ratings received in the third year of medical school. Substantial relationships are shown between the offers of further training and those ratings.

Journal of Medical Education, 1983, *58,* 837–843. https://doi.org/10.1097/00001888-198311000-00001

4.1.10 Cognitive and Noncognitive Factors in Predicting the Clinical Performance of Medical School Graduates

Mohammadreza Hojat, Bette D. Borenstein, and J. Jon Veloski

It is widely believed that both cognitive factors (knowledge, skills, and technical abilities) and noncognitive factors (interpersonal skills, attitudes, and personal qualities) contribute to a physician's competence. With concerns about medical costs being expressed by health professionals, insurance carriers, and public media and with the increased awareness of the psychosocial aspects of good health, the noncognitive elements of medical care deserve the serious attention of healthcare evaluators.

This study was designed to investigate which of these three components of competence (cognitive, noncognitive, or socioeconomic aspects of patient care) contributes most significantly to predicting the performance of residents on an examination of patient management skills (Part III of the National Board Examinations) and to predicting an offer of further residency training by program supervisors. Data were collected on 609 first-year residents who graduated from Jefferson Medical College from 1980 through 1983 and for whom data on postgraduate rating forms were available. The postgraduate rating form consisted of 33 statements that dealt with three aspects of clinical competence: data gathering and processing skills, interpersonal skills and attitudes, and socioeconomic aspects of patient care. An additional question on the form asked whether the supervisor would be willing to offer further training to the graduate.

The correlations between the Part III examination scores and the scores on factor 1 (data gathering and processing skills), factor 2 (interpersonal skills and attitudes), and factor 3 (socioeconomic aspects of patient care) were 0.18 ($p < 0.01$), 0.00, and 0.15 ($p < 0.01$), respectively. Corresponding correlations between being offered further residency training and the three factors were 0.24 ($p < 0.01$), 0.37 ($p < 0.01$), and 0.04, respectively.

Despite the emphasis that has been placed on the cognitive dimensions of clinical competence, the present findings that the noncognitive factor yielded a higher correlation than the cognitive factor with an offer of further residency training indicate that the noncognitive factor was a better predictor than the cognitive. This finding was further supported by obtaining a larger regression weight for the noncognitive factor than the cognitive factor in the multivariate model. The cognitive factor, however, was a statistically significant predictor of the graduates' performance on the Part III examination, which evaluates patient management skills.

Journal of Medical Education, 1988, *63*, 323–325. https://doi.org/10.1097/00001888-198804000-00009

4.1.11 Is the Glass Half Full or Half Empty? A Reexamination of the Associations Between Assessment Measures During Medical School and Clinical Competence After Graduation

Mohammadreza Hojat, Joseph S. Gonnella, J. Jon Veloski, and James B. Erdmann

The purpose of this study was to investigate the associations between performances during medical school and in the first year of residency. It was hypothesized that the strength of such associations is a function of several variables, including similarities of the measured concepts, formats of the assessments, time interval between the assessments, performance levels, and specialty areas. The total sample consisted of 2368 graduates of Jefferson Medical College between 1980 and 1990. The performance measures in medical school were grades on objective examinations in basic and clinical sciences, global ratings of clinical competence in junior core clerkships, and scores on the Part I and Part II examinations of the National Board of Medical Examiners (NBME). The postgraduate performance measures were scores on the Part III NBME examination, postgraduate competence ratings, and board certification. The ratings of postgraduate clinical competence (available for 73% of graduates) were made by residency directors at the end of the first year of residency in the areas of data gathering and processing skills, interpersonal skills and attitudes, and socioeconomic aspects of patient care. Results supported the research hypotheses. It was found that the associations varied for difference measures, at different levels of performance, and in different specialties. The authors conclude that the glass is "half full" regarding the associations between assessment measures before and after graduation from medical school.

Academic Medicine, 1993, *68*(Supplement), S69–S76. https://doi.org/10.1097/00001888-199302000-00035

Also in Gonnella, J.S., Hojat, M., Erdmann, J.B., & Veloski, J.J. (Eds.). (1993). *Assessment measures in medical school, residency and practice: The connections.* (Chapter 14, pp. 137–152). New York: Springer.

4.1.12   Components of Postgraduate Competence: Analyses of 30 Years of Longitudinal Data

Mohammadreza Hojat, David L. Paskin, Clara A. Callahan, Thomas J. Nasca,
Daniel Z. Louis, J. Jon Veloski James B. Erdmann
and Joseph S. Gonnella

Context: The conceptualization and measurement of competence in patient care are critical to the design of medical education programs and outcome assessment.

Objective: We aimed to examine the major components and correlates of postgraduate competence in patient care.

Methods: A 24-item rating form with additional questions about resident doctors' performance and future residency offers was used. Study participants comprised 4560 subjects who graduated from Jefferson Medical College between 1975 and 2004. They pursued their graduate medical education in 508 hospitals. We used a longitudinal study design in which the rating form was completed by program directors to evaluate residents at the end of the first postgraduate year. Factor analysis was used to identify the underlying components of postgraduate ratings. Multiple regression, *t*-test, and correlational analyses were used to study the validity of the components that emerged.

Results: Two major components emerged, which we labeled "Knowledge and Clinical Capabilities" and "Professionalism," and which addressed the science and art of medicine, respectively. Performance measures during medical school, scores on medical licensing examinations, and global assessment of medical knowledge, clinical judgement, and data gathering skills showed higher correlations with scores on the knowledge and clinical capabilities component. Global assessments of professional attitudes and ratings of empathic behavior showed higher correlations with scores on the professionalism component. Offers of continued residency and evaluations of desirable qualities were associated with both components.

Conclusions: Psychometric support for measuring the components of knowledge and clinical capabilities, and professionalism, provides an instrument to empirically evaluate educational outcomes to medical educators who are in search of such a tool.

Medical Education, 2007, *41*(10), 982–989. https://onlinelibrary.wiley.com/doi/10.1111/j.1365-2923.2007.02841.x

4.1.13   Components of Clinical Competence Ratings of Physicians: An Empirical Approach

Mohammadreza Hojat, J. Jon Veloski, and Bette D. Borenstein

The study investigated the underlying structure of ratings of clinical competence. The study sample comprised of 609 physicians graduating from Jefferson Medical College between 1980 and 1983. The rating instrument consisted of 33 statements on clinical behavior in Likert-type format filled out by directors of medical education programs at postgraduate training institutions. The data were subjected to factor analysis. Three factors emerged involving "data gathering and processing skills," "interpersonal and attitudinal," and "socioeconomic" dimensions. Correlations of factor scores with independent measures of conceptually related and unrelated constructs supported the appropriateness of the assigned factor titles. It was concluded that ratings of clinical competence represent a multidimensional construct involving at least three dimensions.

Educational and Psychological Measurement, 1986, *46*, 761–769.

4.1.14   Conceptualization and Measurement of Clinical Competence of Residents: A Brief Rating Form and Its Psychometric Properties

Thomas J. Nasca, Joseph S. Gonnella, Mohammadreza Hojat, J. Jon Veloski, James B. Erdmann, Mary R. Robeson, Timothy P. Brigham, and Clara A. Callahan

Conceptualization and measurement of clinical competence of residents are of interest to medical educators. Yet there is a scarcity of operational tools with satisfactory psychometric support for measuring clinical competence. In this study, we investigated the underlying structure, criterion-related validity, and alpha reliability of a brief rating form (20 items) developed to assess clinical competence of residents. The study sample consisted of 882 physicians (654 men, 228 women) in postgraduate training at Thomas Jefferson University Hospital between 1998 and 2000. Construct validity of the form was supported by factor analysis. Two relevant factors emerged: "knowledge, data gathering, and processing skills" and "interpersonal skills and attitudes." Criterion-related validity was supported by significant linear associates between factor scores and performance on the medical licensing examinations. Alpha reliability coefficients for the two factors were 0.98 and 0.97, respectively. This brief rating form can be employed as one measure to evaluate clinical competence of residents with reasonable confidence in its measurement properties.

Medical Teacher, 2002, *24*(3), 299–303. https://www.tandfonline.com/doi/abs/10.1080/01421590220134141

4.1.15 Relationships Between Performance in Medical School and First Postgraduate Year

*J. Jon Veloski, Mary W. Herman, Joseph S. Gonnella, Carter Zeleznik,
and William F. Kellow*

Changes in medical education have been recommended from both within and without the medical profession because of a growing dissatisfaction with the healthcare system and with the performance of physicians. These recommendations have included modifications of the medical school admission process, the medical curriculum, and the evaluation of prospective medical students.

Data from a longitudinal study of Jefferson Medical College graduates were analyzed to determine the levels of clinical competence in the first postgraduate year and relationships between postgraduate ratings and performance during medical school. Ratings were obtained on knowledge, data gathering skills, clinical judgment, and professional attitudes from the hospitals in which the graduates were receiving their first year's postgraduate training. Significant relationships were found among three levels of performance in medical school and postgraduate ratings in all four competence areas. Relationships were strongest at the highest and lowest performance levels. It was concluded that, in a substantial number of cases, performance in the first postgraduate year could be predicted on the basis of information available to the medical school faculty. It was also concluded that such a monitoring program could provide medical schools with valuable information and clues to possible weaknesses in their educational programs.

Journal of Medical Education, 1979, *54,* 909–916. https://doi.org/10.1097/00001888-197912000-00001

4.1.16   Affirmative Action and Special Consideration Admissions to Medical Education

Jon Veloski, Mohammadreza Hojat, James B. Erdmann, and Joseph S. Gonnella

This is a commentary about a study in which investigators failed to directly investigate affirmative action in underrepresented minority students. Instead, they studied a proxy sample of students who were admitted with low undergraduate GPAs, MCAT scores, or both. Conflicting findings were reported between measures of performance in medical school and outcome measures such as residency ratings, board certification rates, and faculty status that were overlooked by the study authors. A limitation of the study concerns the collecting of postgraduate rating data retrospectively for some graduates more than 20 years after medical school completion with no indication as to how many of the respondents had actually supervised these graduates. Although the study sample performed drastically lower on the medical licensing examinations and their failure rate was six times higher than their classmates, no important difference was detected in their career outcome measures. These findings were found to be inconsistent with our research findings from the Jefferson Longitudinal Study in comparing race and ethnicity. It was suggested that clarification of findings and plausible explanation of differences are needed to support the study conclusions.

Journal of the American Medical Association (Letter to the Editor), 1998, *279*(7), 508–509.

This abstract was written by the book editors.

4.1.17   A Validity Study of Part III of the National Board Examination

J. Jon Veloski, Mohammadreza Hojat, and Joseph S. Gonnella

The purpose of this study was to investigate the validity of Part III of the National Board Examination, a certifying examination of medical knowledge and patient management abilities. The subjects were 1866 first-year resident physicians who graduated from Jefferson Medical College between 1970 and 1984. Statistically significant correlations were found between scores on this examination on the one hand and measures of basic and clinical sciences in medical school and Parts I and II of the National Board Examination on the other hand. Also, graduates who were rated high on supervisors' ratings of clinical competence areas in residency obtained higher scores on the examination than those rated low on this scale even when their baseline knowledge (scores on Part II) was controlled by employing analysis of covariance. In addition, assumptions were made that graduates who were offered further residency training and those who pursued broader, less specialized careers would score higher on this examination. Both assumptions were confirmed. This 15-year study not only provides unique information about the validity of one certifying examination, but it also presents a model that might be used to evaluate other certification tests. Improvements in validity produced by new testing methods, such as computerized administration, could be put into perspective by using similar validity studies.

Evaluation and the Health Professions, 1990, *13*, 227–240.
Copyright© 1990. Sage Publishing. https://journals.sagepub.com/doi/pdf/10.1177/016327879001300206
Also in *Proceedings of the Twenty-Sixth Annual Conference on Research in Medical Education*, Washington, DC. November 1987, 54–59.

4.2   Specialization and Professional Activities

4.2.1   Correlates of Young Physicians' Support for Unionization to Maintain Professional Influence

Virginia U. Collier, Mohammadreza Hojat, Susan L. Rattner, Joseph S. Gonnella, James B. Erdmann, Thomas J. Nasca, and J. Jon Veloski

Purpose: Given the recent approval of a resolution in support of physician unionization by the AMA House of Delegates, it is timely to empirically investigate the factors associated with physicians' approval of unionization. This study was designed to investigate correlates of young physicians' support for unionization.

Method: A survey was mailed to all 1987–1992 Jefferson Medical College graduates (*n* = 1272); 835 (66%) responded.

Results: Forty-three percent of young physicians supported, 31% did not support unionization, and 26% expressed no opinion. Surgeons, medical subspecialists, pediatricians, and hospital-based specialists were more likely to support unionization than family physicians. Significant predictors of unionization support were negative views of the changes in the healthcare system, negative perceptions of the quality of care provided by managed care, and beliefs that physicians' independence had been impaired by changes in the healthcare system and that physicians' personal satisfaction should take precedence over societal needs in determining the future of health care. Support for unionization also correlated with physicians' perceptions that mental health patients should be referred to psychiatrists, that physician-assisted suicide should be legalized, and that the involvement of nurse practitioners in diagnosis and treatment could compromise the quality of care. Support for unionization was unrelated to gender, academic achievement, performance on licensing examinations, ratings of clinical competence, and educational debt.

Conclusions: Young physician support for unionization is a function of frustration with market-driven policies that compromise the quality of care and negatively affect physician autonomy and personal satisfaction.

Academic Medicine, 2001, *76*(10), 1039–1044.   https://doi.org/10.1097/00001888-200110000-00014

4.2.2   Stability and Change of Interest in Obstetrics-Gynecology Among Medical Students: 18 Years of Longitudinal Data

Iraj Forouzan and Mohammadreza Hojat

The purpose was to compare the percentage of students who maintain interest in specializing in obstetrics-gynecology during medical school with the percentages of students maintaining interest in other selected specialties, and to examine changes of interest from obstetrics-gynecology to other specialties and from other specialties to obstetrics-gynecology. A longitudinal cohort study comparing the stability of students' interests in obstetrics-gynecology and in other specialties was performed by using data on 2889 graduates of 18 classes of Jefferson Medical College of Thomas Jefferson University between 1975 and 1992. The percentage of students who maintained interest in obstetrics-gynecology, as measured at the beginning and end of medical school, was 19%, compared with 40% for internal medicine and surgery, 39% for family medicine, and 22% for pediatrics. By the time they graduated, some students who had planned as freshman to pursue obstetrics-gynecology had changed their interests to internal medicine (19%), surgery (17%), family medicine (8%), or pediatrics (7%). In turn, obstetrics-gynecology attracted students who had initially expressed interest in other specialties: 17% from family medicine, 14% from surgery, 12% from internal medicine, and 8% from pediatrics. Despite the low percentage of students who maintained interest in obstetrics-gynecology, the overall percentage of students interested in obstetrics-gynecology at the time of graduation was somewhat greater than the percentage of students interested at the start of medical school. That only about one-fifth of the students initially interested in obstetrics-gynecology maintained their interest, and that many students' interest changed from one specialty to another, suggests that factors contributing to changes in interest need further investigation.

Academic Medicine, 1993, *68*, 919–922. https://journals.lww.com/academicmedicine/Abstract/1993/12000/Stability_and_change_of_interest_in.13.aspx

4.2.3   Medical Education and Health Services Research: The Linkage

Joseph S. Gonnella, Clara A. Callahan, Daniel Z. Louis, Mohammadreza Hojat, and James B. Erdmann

The medical community is coming under increased scrutiny. Challenges to the integrity of the healthcare system have been raised due to reports about the prevalence of medical errors. A heightened level of vigilance is required. Equally important is the need to isolate and correct the source of any problem, perceived or real. We are faced with challenging questions: Is the selection of students and residents appropriate? Are their education and evaluation valid? These questions must be answered at least in part by understanding the climate in which the services to the patients are rendered. Otherwise, deficiencies noted in practice may be inappropriately attributed to the educational process. This article addresses the importance, implications, and impact of the link between medical education and health services research. The goal of medical education is to prepare physicians to meet the challenges of practice by fulfilling their roles of clinician, educator, and resource manager. Health services research can be linked to any of these physician roles. An understanding of health services is necessary to assess how well this goal is being met in the context of the changing healthcare system. A partnership between medical education and health services research is essential for academic health centers and health services institutions in assessing issues of health manpower and for the public good. Academic health centers have an important role in this partnership providing an infrastructure and expertise for both education and health services research.

Medical Teacher (Editorial), 2004, *26*(1), 7–11. https://www.tandfonline.com/doi/abs/10.1080/0142159032000156515

4.2.4 The Impact of Early Career Specialization on Licensing Requirements and Related Educational Implications

Joseph S. Gonnella, Mohammadreza Hojat, James B. Erdmann, and J. Jon Veloski

Purpose: It was hypothesized that physicians who pursue early career specialization in their first year of graduate medical education after medical school are likely to experience a decline in their scores on the medical licensing examination.

Method: A longitudinal prospective design was used in which 1927 physicians who graduated from Jefferson Medical College between 1980 and 1991 were studied. Type of first-year graduate training program was the independent variable, and performance on a medical licensing examination (Part III examination of the National Board of Medical Examiners [NBME]) was the dependent variable. Scores of Parts I and II of the NBME taken in medical school, medical school class rank, and gender were the control variables.

Results: Findings showed significant differences on Part III scores among physicians in 12 different graduate programs despite statistical adjustments for baseline differences. Physicians in family medicine and emergency medicine programs obtained the highest adjusted Part III scores, followed by physicians in internal medicine and transitional programs. The next group consisted of physicians in pediatrics, obstetrics-gynecology, anesthesiology, and general surgery programs. The group with the lowest Part III scores included physicians in pathology, radiology, and psychiatry.

Implications: These findings suggest that students who meet only the minimal standards in medical school should be advised to pursue a broad training program in the first year of graduate medical education to strengthen their general clinical competence as a means to increase their chances of passing licensing examinations.

Advances in Health Sciences Education, 1996, *1*(2), 125–139.

4.2.5   The Impact of Early Specialization on the Clinical Competence of Residents

Joseph S. Gonnella and J. Jon Veloski

To study the relation between first-year postgraduate training and performance on a test of general clinical competence, we analyzed results on the Part III National Board Examination according to the type of residency chosen by 1514 graduates of Jefferson Medical College between 1970 and 1979. The results show that physicians in family medicine, internal medicine, or flexible programs score higher on Part III than do those in surgery, pediatrics, obstetrics-gynecology, psychiatry, or pathology, even after correction for their performance on Part II of the boards. Although these differences could be due to other factors, we suggest that in the first year of some residency programs, knowledge and skills in broad areas of medicine are not being sufficiently emphasized, and that changes are needed to strengthen the residents' general capabilities.

The New England Journal of Medicine, 1982, *306*, 275–277.

Also in *Proceedings of the Nineteenth Annual Conference on Research in Medical Education*, Washington, DC. November 1980, 142–147.

4.2.6   Should Half of All Medical School Graduates Enter Primary Care? Perceptions of Faculty Members at Jefferson Medical College

Jonathan Gottlieb, Sylvia K. Fields, Mohammadreza Hojat, and J. Jon Veloski

Purpose: This study was undertaken to promote communication among faculty regarding the impact of a proposed goal that 50% of the graduates of Jefferson Medical College enter generalist careers. Since the opinions and attitudes of faculty regarding career decisions may directly or indirectly influence students, the authors investigated faculty's views of the optimal ratio of primary care to non-primary care physicians in the workforce and their perceptions of the effect on medical education, research, and healthcare delivery if the 50% goal were to be mandated.

Method: A questionnaire was mailed in January 1994 to all 694 salaried faculty of Jefferson Medical College. Respondents' opinions about the optimal primary care to non-primary care ratio and their perceptions of the effects of implementing the 50% goal on 21 areas related to medical education, research, and healthcare delivery were examined using a Likert-type scale. Obstacles perceived by non-primary care physicians as preventing their practice of primary care were also among the outcome measures.

Results: A total of 275 completed questionnaires were received (40% response rate; 72 primary care physicians, 141 non-primary care physicians, and 62 nonphysicians). The median and mode of an optimal primary care-to-non-primary care ratio were both 50/50. Faculty, in general, perceived that implementing the 50% goal would enhance public access to primary care, physician-patient relationships, utilization of nonphysicians, and career satisfaction of generalists. They predicted decreases in costs of care, freedom of career choice, funding, and interest in research. The primary care physicians perceived greater enhancements of the image of physicians, quality of care, and satisfaction of generalists and subspecialists than did the non-primary care physicians. Gender and age did not affect the perceptions. A lack of appropriate training was identified by 45% and a lack of interest by 28% of the non-primary care physicians as major obstacles to their practice of primary care medicine.

Conclusion: The faculty members' positive and negative views of the proposed reform can provide useful information to the institution in understanding the potential impediments to increasing the numbers of generalist graduates. The generalists had significantly different views from the subspecialists about the impact of increasing the proportion of primary care physicians on healthcare delivery and research. In general the primary care physicians were more likely to view the proposed changes as beneficial than the non-primary care physicians.

Academic Medicine, 1995, *70*, 1125–1133.   https://pubmed.ncbi.nlm.nih.gov/7495458/

4.2.7 *Family Medicine and Primary Care: Trends and Student Characteristics*

Mary W. Herman and J. Jon Veloski

Using data from a longitudinal study of medical students at Jefferson Medical College, the authors analyzed trends in senior student interest in primary care specialties between 1971 and 1975 and selected background characteristics and performance levels of students choosing family medicine compared with those in other specialties. The study demonstrated a rising trend in the proportion of Jefferson seniors interested in family practice but not in internal medicine or pediatrics. Unlike the medical graduates entering general practice in earlier years, students interested in family medicine performed as well or better than those in all other specialties except internal medicine. Differences in the academic performance between students interested in internal medicine and family medicine remained even when only those interested primarily in clinical careers were compared. The proportion of students interested in family medicine residencies increased from 6% to 17% in the study period. Smaller proportions were interested in teaching and research than those in other specialties, and larger proportions intended to work in communities with populations of 100,000 or less.

Journal of Medical Education, 1977, *52*, 99–106. https://doi.org/10.1097/00001888-197702000-00002

4.2.8 Primary Care and Non-primary Care Physicians: A Longitudinal Study of Their Similarities, Differences, and Correlates Before, During, and After Medical School

Mohammadreza Hojat, Joseph S. Gonnella, James B. Erdmann, J. Jon Veloski, and Gang Xu

Purpose: To investigate similarities and differences between physicians in primary care and non-primary care specialties on performance measures prior to, during, and after medical school, and on demographic characteristics, professional plans and preferences in medical school, professional activities, career satisfaction, perceived problems, and research activities, and to predict primary-non-primary care career choices from information obtained in medical school.

Method: A questionnaire was mailed to 1076 physicians who graduated from Jefferson Medical College between 1982 and 1986. Of those who responded (62%), 232 were primary care and 406 were non-primary care physicians (29 physicians in mixed specialties were excluded). Data from the questionnaire concerning professional activities, satisfaction, problems, and research productivities were merged with the college's longitudinal study database.

Results: Comparisons of primary care-non-primary care physicians indicated no significant difference between them on performance measures before, during, and after medical school, with the exception that non-primary care physicians had higher scores on quantitative tests before medical school, and primary care physicians scored higher on a licensing examination of general clinical skills and patient management taken during residency training. Also, compared with non-primary care physicians, those in primary care were less likely to be employed full-time, were less likely to locate in metropolitan areas, had a lower rate of academic appointment, and had a higher rate of board certification. Other results showed differences between the groups in terms of age at entrance to medical school, proportion of women, estimates during medical school of anticipated income, career plans during medical school, satisfaction with career and income, and research and scientific activities.

A logistic regression model could predict primary care-non-primary care status from specialty interest, professional plans, and interests expressed in medical school.

Academic Medicine, 1995, *70*(Supplement): S17–S28. https://doi.org/10.1097/00001888-199501000-00020

4.2.9 Differences in Professional Activities, Perceptions of Professional Problems, and Practice Patterns Between Men and Women Graduates of Jefferson Medical College

Mohammadreza Hojat, Joseph S. Gonnella, J. Jon Veloski, and Shelley L. Moses

Differences between men and women graduates of one medical school in practice patterns, professional activities, and problems were investigated. A questionnaire was mailed in 1986 to 600 physicians, randomly selected from 1102 who had graduated from Jefferson Medical College of Thomas Jefferson University between 1977 and 1981. Four hundred and fifty (364 men and 86 women) responded (75%). The women were less likely than the men to be employed full-time; however, proportionately more women than men held full-time academic appointments, treated patients from low-income families, and served in underserved areas in inner cities. The women reported working fewer hours per week and having fewer patients than did the men. The women published scientific articles as often as did the men but were less likely to serve on professional committees, receive professional awards, or develop medical procedures. The women were less concerned about the oversupply of physicians and malpractice litigation. Implications of the findings for health manpower planning and practice pattern expectations are discussed.

Academic Medicine, 1990, *65*, 755–761. https://doi.org/10.1097/0000 1888-199012000-00011
   Also in *Proceedings of the Twenty-Sixth Annual Conference on Research in Medical Education*, Washington, DC. November 1987, 23–27.

4.2.10 A Program to Increase the Number of Family Physicians in Rural and Underserved Areas: Impact After 22 Years

Howard K. Rabinowitz, James J. Diamond, Fred W. Markham,
and Christina E. Hazelwood

Context: The shortage of physicians in rural areas is a long-standing and serious problem, and national and state policymakers and educators continue to face the challenge of finding effective ways to increase the supply of rural physicians.

Objective: To determine the direct and long-term impact of the Physician Shortage Area Program (PSAP) of Jefferson Medical College (JMC) on the rural physician workforce.

Design: Retrospective cohort study.

Participants and Setting: A total of 206 PSAP graduates from the classes of 1978–1991.

Main Outcome Measures: The PSAP graduates currently practicing family medicine in rural and underserved areas of Pennsylvania, compared with all allopathic medical school graduates in the state and with all US and international allopathic graduates. All PSAP graduates were also compared with their non-PSAP peers at JMC regarding their US practice location, medical specialty, and retention for the past 5–10 years.

Results: The PSAP graduates account for 21% (32/150) of family physicians practicing in rural Pennsylvania who graduated from one of the state's seven medical schools, even though they represent only 1% (206/14,710) of graduates from those schools (relative risk [RR], 19.1). Among all US and international medical school graduates, PSAP graduates represent 12% of all family physicians in rural Pennsylvania. Results were similar for PSAP graduates practicing in underserved areas. Overall, PSAP graduates were much more likely than their non-PSAP classmates at JMC to practice in a rural area of the USA (34% vs. 11%; RR, 3.0), to practice in an underserved area (30% vs. 9%; RR, 3.2), to practice family medicine (52% vs. 13%; RR, 4.0), and to have combined a career in family practice with practice in a rural area (21% vs. 2%; RR, 8.5). Of PSAP graduates, 84% were practicing in either a rural or a small metropolitan area, or one of the primary care specialties. Program retention has remained high, with the number of PSAP graduates currently practicing rural family medicine equal to 87% of those practicing between 5 and 10 years ago, and the number practicing in underserved areas, 94%.

Conclusions: The PSAP, after more than 22 years, has had a disproportionately large impact on the rural physician workforce, and this effect has persisted over time. Based on these program results, policymakers and medical schools can have a substantial impact on the shortage of physicians in rural areas.

Reprinted with permission from *Journal of the American Medical Association*, 1999, *281*(3), 255–260.

4.2.11   Critical Factors for Designing Programs to Increase the Supply and Retention of Rural Primary Care Physicians

Howard K. Rabinowitz, James J. Diamond, Fred W. Markham,
and Nina P. Paynter

Context: The Physician Shortage Area Program (PSAP) of Jefferson Medical College (Philadelphia, PA) is one of a small number of medical school programs that address the shortage of rural primary care physicians. However, little is known regarding why these programs work.

Objectives: To identify factors independently predictive of rural primary care supply and retention and to determine which components of the PSAP lead to its outcomes.

Design: Retrospective cohort study.

Setting and Participants: A total of 3414 Jefferson Medical College graduates from the classes of 1978–1993, including 220 PSAP graduates.

Main Outcome Measures: Rural primary care practice and retention in 1999 as predicted by 19 previously collected variables. Twelve variables were available for all classes; 7 variables were collected only for 1978–1982 graduates.

Results: Freshman-year plan for family practice, being in the PSAP, having a National Health Service Corps scholarship, male sex, and taking an elective senior family practice rural preceptorship (the only factor not available at entrance to medical school) were independently predictive of physicians practicing rural primary care. For 1978–1982 graduates, growing up in a rural area was the only additionally collected independent predictor of rural primary care (odds ratio [OR], 4.0; 95% CI, 2.1–7.6; $p < 0.001$). Participation in the PSAP was the only independent predictive factor of retention for all classes (OR, 4.7; 95% CI, 2.0–11.2; $p < 0.001$). Among PSAP graduates, taking a senior rural preceptorship was independently predictive of rural primary care (OR, 2.5; 95% CI, 1.3–4.7; $p = 0.004$). However, non-PSAP graduates with two key selection characteristics of PSAP students (having grown up in a rural area and freshman-year plans for family practice) were 78% as likely as PSAP graduates to be rural primary care physicians, and 75% as likely to remain, suggesting that the admissions component of the PSAP is the most important reason for its success. In fact, few graduates without either of these factors were rural primary care physicians (1.8%).

Conclusions: Medical educators and policymakers can have the greatest impact on the supply and retention of rural primary care physicians by developing programs to increase the number of medical school matriculants with background and career plans that make them most likely to pursue these career goals. Curricular experiences and other factors can further increase these outcomes, especially by supporting those already likely to become rural primary care physicians.

Reprinted with permission from *Journal of the American Medical Association*, 2001, *286*(9), 1041–1048.

4.2.12   Who Is a Generalist? An Analysis of Whether Physicians Trained as Generalists Practice as Generalists

Howard K. Rabinowitz, Mohammadreza Hojat, J. Jon Veloski, Susan L. Rattner, Mary R. Robeson, Gang Xu, Marilyn H. Appel, Carol Cochran, Robert L. Jones, and Steven L. Kanter

Accurate data on the number of generalist physicians are needed to monitor the physician workforce and to plan for future requirements in the changing healthcare system. This study assessed the relationship between two frequently used definitions of a generalist physician: completion of graduate medical education (GME) in only a generalist discipline and physician's self-report of practicing as a generalist. Data for 4808 physician graduates from six Pennsylvania medical schools from 1986 to 1991 were analyzed using information from the GME tracking census of the Association of American Medical Colleges and the Physician Masterfile of the American Medical Association. Of 1291 physicians trained in a generalist discipline, 1205 (93%) reported practicing as generalists. Conversely, of the 3517 not trained in a generalist discipline, 3358 (95%) were not practicing as generalists. These results indicate that GME training is a valid predictor of self-reported practice and provide baseline data to monitor future changes.

Evaluation & The Health Profession, 1999, 22, 539–544.

4.2.13   A Statewide System to Track Medical Students' Careers: The Pennsylvania Model

*Howard K. Rabinowitz, J. Jon Veloski, Robert C. Aber, Sheldon Adler,
Silvia Ferretti, Gerald J. Kelliher, Eugene Mochen, Gail Morrison,
Susan L. Rattner, Gerald Sterling, Mary R. Robeson, Mohammadreza Hojat,
and Gang Xu*

In 1994 the Commonwealth of Pennsylvania announced a statewide Generalist Physician Initiative (GPI) modeled after the Robert Wood Johnson Foundation's GPI. Three-year grants totaling more than $9 million were awarded to seven of Pennsylvania's medical schools, including two that had already received GPI grants from the foundation. Stimulated by these initiatives, the state's six allopathic and two osteopathic medical schools decided to work together to develop a collaborative longitudinal tracking system to follow the careers of all their students from matriculation into their professional careers. This statewide data system, which includes information for more than 18,000 students and graduates beginning with the entering class of 1982, can be used to evaluate the impact of the Pennsylvania GPI, and it also yielded a local longitudinal tracking system for each medical school. This paper outlines the concept of the system, its technical implementation, and the corresponding implications for other medical schools considering the development of similar outcome assessment systems.

Academic Medicine, 1999, *74*(January Supplement), S112–S118. https://doi.org/10.1097/00001888-199901001-00042

4.2.14 Generalist Career Plans: Tracking Medical School Seniors Through Residency

Howard K. Rabinowitz, Gang Xu, Mary R. Robeson, Mohammadreza Hojat, Susan L. Rattner, Marilyn H. Appel, Carol Cochran, Jeffrey J. Johnson, Steven L. Kanter, and J. Jon Veloski

Context: Public and private groups undertaking initiatives to increase the number of generalist physicians require systematic data to assess the outcomes of their efforts. In particular, information about the consistency between generalist career plans at the end of medical school and completion of residency is lacking.

Method: Senior career plans as reported on the AAMC GQ and subsequent outcomes at the end of graduate medical education were studied for 2530 physicians who graduated from six Pennsylvania medical schools in 1990–1992.

Results: Overall, 24% of the seniors planned generalist careers and 27% left their residency in family practice, internal medicine, or pediatrics without subspecializing. Of the seniors planning to be generalists, 86% maintained that direction throughout graduate medical education.

Conclusion: The aggregate results of seniors' career plans are reasonably accurate predictors of career direction at the end of graduate medical education. However, as medical schools, foundations, and government agencies monitor the results of their generalists' initiatives, it is now clear that assessment must be based not only on students' intentions at the end of medical school and early in residency, but also on career decisions throughout graduate medical education.

Academic Medicine, 1997, 72, 103–105.   https://doi.org/10.1097/00001888-199710001-00035

4.2.15   Choice of First-Year Residency Position and Long-Term Generalist Career Choices

Howard K. Rabinowitz, Gang Xu, J. Jon Veloski, Susan L. Rattner,
Mary R. Robeson, Mohammadreza Hojat, Marilyn H. Apple, Carol Cochran,
Robert L. Jones, and Steven L. Kanter

The most commonly used annual indicator of primary care outcomes has been the percentage of medical school graduates enrolled in first-year graduate medical education programs in three generalist disciplines of family medicine, internal medicine, and pediatrics. Little information is available regarding the accuracy of first-year residency specialty choice in predicting subsequent primary care practice. However, since the rates of subspecialization differ across the three generalist disciplines, summing up the number of physicians entering generalist programs in the first year of postgraduate medical education to estimate the future supply of primary care physicians is likely to be inaccurate. In this study of 2548 medical school graduates from the classes of 1990–1992 at six Pennsylvania medical schools, we obtained information from the AAMC regarding each graduate's first-year residency program, their career plan reported on the graduation questionnaire completed in the last year of medical school, and residency specialty at the completion of the graduate medical education training. We found that 27% of the graduates in the study sample completed their graduate medical education training in primary care (which had been highly correlated with self-reported practice specialty). By following a cohort of graduates from the study sample, we found that beginning a residency in each of the three generalist disciplines was associated with very different likelihood of pursuing a career in primary care. For example, 100% of those entering first-year residency programs in family medicine continued as generalists, compared with 52% for internal medicine, and 73% for pediatrics. Thus, merely adding the number of graduates entering first-year programs in the three primary care disciplines to estimate generalist outcomes results in a substantial overestimate of the number of actual generalists.

Journal of the American Medical Association (Letter to the Editor), 2000, *284*(9), 1081–1082.
This abstract was written by the book editors.

4.2.16 Assessment of Physicians' Interest in Primary Care Training/Retraining

Susan L. Rattner, Mary R. Robeson, and J. Jon Veloski

Purpose: To assess generalists' and specialists' interest in primary care training and the factors associated with this interest.

Method: The study sample was drawn from the alumni of the Jefferson Medical College of Thomas Jefferson University (classes of 1970–1990) who were practicing in Pennsylvania. Family practitioners and general internists were defined as generalists; obstetrician-gynecologists (ob-gyns) and internal medicine subspecialists were defined as specialists. In 1995 a questionnaire was mailed consisting of 46 items assessing the physicians' interest in participating in primary care educational programs, reasons for any such interest, and preferences for content. Two items on the specialists' questionnaire asked about changing careers from specialist to generalist, and two items on the generalists' questionnaire asked about broadening the scope of their practices.

Results: The response rate was 54% (381/707). In all, 78% of the physicians expressed interest in primary care training. The generalists were more interested in primary care training than were the specialists ($p < 0.001$). The ob-gyns were more interested in primary care training than were the medical subspecialists ($p = 0.01$). Few of the medical subspecialists and no ob-gyns were influenced by plans to change careers to primary care. More of the ob-gyns than the medical subspecialists were motivated by plans to shift emphasis to provide more primary care.

Conclusion: The results suggest (1) that although many specialists have an interest in primary care training, it is rarely motivated by plans to change to primary care practice, and (2) that generalists are very interested in expanding their abilities. Both of these findings should be considered in workforce planning.

Academic Medicine, 1997, 72, 1103–1105. https://doi.org/10.1097/00001888-199712000-00023

4.2.17   Changing Specialties: Do Anesthesiologists Differ from Other Physicians?

Joseph L. Seltzer and J. Jon Veloski

Data for the present study were derived from a longitudinal study of medical students and graduates conducted at Jefferson Medical College since 1968. Questionnaires were available for 1306 (78%) of the 1676 students in the graduating classes of 1968 through 1976. The actual specialties of all but 155 of these Jefferson graduates were obtained 5 or more years after graduation from the alumni office of the College. The remaining 1151 (69%) graduates were classified into 11 large specialty groupings and 1 group that included small numbers of graduates in ophthalmology, otolaryngology, and preventive medicine programs. Thirty-five (3%) of the 1151 graduates listed anesthesiology as their specialty. Of the 31 students who had planned, prior to graduation, to go into anesthesiology, 26 actually did so. Nine physicians had changes from other specialties to anesthesiology, which represented a 26% gain. It was concluded from the study that, for whatever reasons physicians change specialties, anesthesiology does not appear to be different from other specialties in its ability to retain or gain physicians. The data in this study represent only one medical school and, if students at other medical colleges receive different types or amounts of formal training in anesthesiology, there could be a greater number of physicians changing to or from anesthesiology.

Anesthesia and Analgesia, 1982, *61*(6), 504–506.

4.2.18   Migration of Physicians to and from Anesthesiology

Joseph L. Seltezer and Jon Veloski

This letter calls attention to the value of prospective longitudinal studies when investigating young physicians' career paths during residency education. A researcher using retrospective career path data from the graduates of multiple medical schools had reported patterns of changes in specialty choice during residency that differed from findings reported in an earlier Jefferson study. The author attributed this discrepancy, in part, to the limitation of the Jefferson study to a single medical school.

Seltzer and Veloski penned this letter to the editor to assert that a prospective longitudinal plan for data collection on changes in career path from medical school through residency over multiple graduating classes can yield more valid findings and compensate for the limitation of a single school.

Anesthesia and Analgesia (Letter to the Editor), 1983, *62*, 702. https://journals.lww. com/anesthesia-analgesia/Citation/1983/01000/Migration_of_Physicians_to_and_ from_Anesthesiology.27.aspx

This abstract was written by the book editors.

4.2.19   Academic Performance of Psychiatrists Compared to Other Specialists Before, During, and After Medical School

Frederick S. Sierles, Michael J. Vergare, Mohammadreza Hojat, and Joseph S. Gonnella

Objective: This study was designed to compare psychiatrists with other physicians on measures of academic performance before, during, and after medical school.

Method: More than three decades of data for graduates of Jefferson Medical College ($N = 5701$) were analyzed. Those who pursued psychiatry were compared to physicians in seven other specialties on 18 performance measures. Analysis of covariance was used to control for gender effect.

Results: Compared to other physicians, psychiatrists scored higher on measures of verbal ability and general information before medical school and on evaluations of knowledge and skills in behavioral sciences during medical school, but they scored lower on the United States Medical Licensing Examination, Step 3.

Conclusions: The results generally confirmed the authors' expectations about psychiatrists' academic performance. More attention should be paid to the general medical education of psychiatrists.

American Journal of Psychiatry, 2004, *161*(8), 1477–1482. https://ajp.psychiatry-online.org/doi/full/10.1176/appi.ajp.161.8.1477

4.2.20   Board Certification in Obstetrics and Gynecology: Associations with Physicians' Demographics and Performances During Medical School

Cynthia G. Silber and J. Jon Veloski

Objective: This study was undertaken to investigate the relationship of demographics, medical school performance, and licensing examination scores to board certification.

Study Design: A longitudinal follow-up study of graduates of Jefferson Medical College between 1968 and 1994 identified in the AMA Physicians' Professional Data (AMA-PPD) file as practicing obstetrics and gynecology in 2003. Demographics, grades, and licensing examination scores had been collected prospectively. Board certification status was obtained from the AMA-PPD in 2003. Bivariate differences were evaluated with t-tests. Logistic regression was used to evaluate multivariate relationships to board certification status.

Results: Of 310 physicians in obstetrics and gynecology, 291 (94%) were board certified. Those without certification were more likely to be underrepresented minorities, to have been older in medical school, and to have weaker academic records. Logistic regression indicated that scores on Step 2 of the United States Medical Licensing Examination were the single most important predictor of achieving board certification. Those with scores of 200 or higher were 7 times more likely to achieve certification than those below 200.

Conclusion: Age, gender, and minority status are not independent predictors of achieving board certification. A low score on the United States Medical Licensing Examination, Step 2, is a risk factor for not achieving certification.

American Journal of Obstetrics and Gynecology, 2005, *192*, 318–322.
Reprinted with permission from Elsevier.

4.2.21   *Performance on the NBME Part II Examination and Career Choice*

Tennyson Williams, Larry Sachs, and J. Jon Veloski

In this study the authors hypothesized that the NBME Part II examination subtest scores of students selecting various specialty residency programs would demonstrate profiles that were unique for each specialty chosen. The hypothesis was based on the assumption that students will seek careers dealing with content with which they are comfortable and that this comfort derives from successful academic performance.

Separate but parallel analyses were conducted on data from the Jefferson Medical College (JMC) and the Ohio State University College of Medicine (OSU). Students from each school who took the NBME Part II Examination from 1978 through 1984 were grouped according to their residency choice: family medicine, internal medicine, obstetrics-gynecology, pediatrics, psychiatry, surgery, and "other." The sample sizes totaled 1534 for JMC and 1429 for OSU.

One of the major results was the similarity of profiles across the two schools. The students who selected a residency for which there was a major subtest in the NBME Part II examination showed a higher performance on the subtest corresponding to their residency choice than on any other subtest. The family medicine group and the "other" group did not have any subtest means significantly different than the group mean. The magnitude of the difference between scores on the subtest of the specialty chosen and other subtests is impressive. The authors consider that counseling to enter particular specialties for students who have scores unusually high on one subtest would be appropriate. Even when a student scores very high on two subtests, the career decisions are made easier. In such cases, students should give high priority to personal factors in deciding between the two disciplines.

Journal   of   Medical   Education,   1986,   *61,*   979–981.   https://doi.org/10.1097/00001888-198612000-00006

4.2.22 Medical Students Who Enter General Surgery Residency Programs: A Follow-Up Between 1972 and 1986

Philip J. Wolfson, Mary R. Robeson, and J. Jon Veloski

It is generally assumed that most students who enter surgical residency programs each year are destined for careers in the surgical field—general surgery, a specialty of general surgery, or a related specialty (ENT, orthopedic surgery, ophthalmology, or urology). While it has always been recognized that a small number of surgical residents do leave the surgical field, little has been reported about what actually happens to them. We undertook this long-term follow-up of our graduates to find out what proportion do end up in a surgical field and to identify any patterns of change that may have taken place over the past 15 years. Between 1972 and 1986, 459 JMC graduates (about 14%) entered PGY-1 programs in general surgery. Using recent follow-up data available from the College's alumni office and the American Medical Association, we classified each of the graduates into one of the three groups: (1) those remaining in general surgery/subspecialty, (2) graduates in a specialty within the surgical field, and (3) those in a specialty outside of the surgical field (anesthesiology, dermatology, family practice, emergency medicine, pediatrics, pathology, or radiology). The three groups were compared across years on demographics, academic credentials, and surgery program director's ratings of their performance in PGY-1.

Throughout the 15-year time period, approximately 70% of the graduates did remain in general surgery/subspecialty while about 15% moved to one of the other specialties within the surgical field. Although the percentage of surgery residents who left the surgical field remained constant throughout nearly two decades, there were statistically significant changes in the academic credentials of the residents who remained within the surgical field compared with those who left. During the mid-1970s the residents who remained within the surgical field had better academic credentials on average as measured by medical school grades and National Board scores (about 40 points higher) than those who switched out of the surgical field. However, in the more recent time period of the late 1970s and the early 1980s, the trend reversed. Those residents who left the surgical field had academic credentials that were, on average, equal to or better than those who remained. There were no differences between the groups on age, sex, and program director's ratings of their performance in the first year of the surgical residency.

These results have important implications for student counseling and resident selection. They suggest that some good students are being recruited into surgical programs but are later being lost in major career switches. Studies need to be undertaken to find out why these students are changing. Perhaps these changes are related to young residents' preferences for specialties that offer more controllable lifestyles than the surgical field.

The American Journal of Surgery, 1991, *162*(5), 491–494.
Reprinted with permission from Elsevier.

4.2.23   Perceptions of Practice Problems Encountered by Family Physicians, Pediatricians, and Orthopedic Surgeons

Gang Xu, Timothy P. Brigham, J. Jon Veloski, and Joseph F. Rodgers

Information about physicians' practice problems was solicited through a structured questionnaire mailed to a group of family physicians, pediatricians, and orthopedic surgeons. Overall, a lack of personal time was the major concern across the three groups of physicians. Comparisons among the three types of physicians revealed two patterns: Family physicians reported more concerns in the "interpersonal" dimension, whereas orthopedic surgeons had more concerns in the "legal-economic" dimension. These patterns of differences persisted with two variables controlled: gender and time period in which they completed their residency program. These findings indicate that physicians' concerns in their practice vary among the special-ties, and they imply that the changed economy and reimbursement system might have more impact on one than the other. Thus the effectiveness of residency training and continuing education might be improved by emphasizing the specialty-related problems in practice.

Evaluation & The Health Professions, 1993, *16*, 119–129.

4.2.24   Primary Care and Non-primary Care Physicians' Concerns in Practice and Perceptions of Medical School Curriculum

Gang Xu, Mohammadreza Hojat, Timothy P. Brigham, Mary R. Robeson, and J. Jon Veloski

The purpose of this study is to address the issue of physicians' concerns in practice and their perception of a medical school's curriculum with an emphasis on comparisons between primary and non-primary care physicians. The sample consisted of 663 physicians who graduated from Jefferson Medical College (JMC) between 1982 and 1986 and also responded to a mailed questionnaire. Comparisons were made between physicians in primary care ($n = 235$) and in non-primary care ($n = 429$) specialties on their responses regarding concerns in medical practice and evaluation of the medical school curriculum. Primary care physicians were more concerned about the time for their professional development whereas non-primary care physicians were more concerned about an oversupply of physicians in their specialties, prospective hospital payment, and malpractice litigation. Regardless of the specialties, the physicians overall seemed very concerned about their personal time. Interpersonal skills were regarded by all respondents as an important aspect of the medical school's curriculum. The importance of psychological, social, and cultural factors in the curriculum was strongly supported by these physicians' responses, particularly among primary care and women physicians.

Evaluation and The Health Professions, 1994, *17*, 436–445.

4.2.25   Factors Associated with Changing Levels of Interest in Primary Care During Medical School

Gang Xu, Mohammadreza Hojat, Timothy P. Brigham, and J. Jon Veloski

Background: Previous studies have indicated that there is a need for an understanding of the effect of medical school curricula on students' choice of primary care specialties. This study examined students' change of interest in primary care as related to their clinical experience during medical school and to other variables.

Method: A total of 1911 (74%) responded to a national survey of all allopathic medical school graduates in early 1993. Their reported change of interest in primary care during medical school was cross-tabulated with their clinical experiences in medical school, their demographics, their interest prior to medical school, and their future plan in practice.

Results: Students' increased interest in primary care during medical school was strongly associated with the electives they took in primary care. The positive change of interest in primary care is also associated with their interest prior to medical school and their future plan in primary care in later career.

Conclusion: Schools wishing to implement a program to increase the number of graduates entering primary care specialties may consider increasing the number of primary care elective courses to increase students' interests and help them make a decision to enter and remain in primary care specialties.

*Academic   Medicine,   1999,   74,   1011–1015.   https://doi.org/10.1097/00001888-199909000-00015

4.2.26 Emergency Medicine Career Change: Associations with Performances in Medical School and in the First Postgraduate Year and with Indebtedness

Gang Xu, Mohammadreza Hojat, and J. Jon Veloski

Objective: Emergency medicine has been identified as the specialty that has gained the most young physicians who have changed their careers. To identify factors that may have contributed to such career changes, the authors compared the characteristics of three groups of physicians trained at their medical school: those who chose and stayed in emergency medicine, those who migrated into emergency medicine from other specialties, and those who moved out of emergency medicine.

Methods: A prospective longitudinal study was conducted. The sample consisted of physicians who chose emergency medicine as their careers at graduation and stayed in the specialty ($n = 24$), those who migrated from other specialties into emergency medicine ($n = 51$), and those who moved out of emergency medicine ($n = 10$). This sample was obtained from a total of 2173 graduates of Jefferson Medical College between 1978 and 1987. The three groups of physicians were compared according to their academic performances both during medical school and after graduation. The dependent variables were freshman and sophomore grade-point averages (GPAs), written clinical examination scores, scores on National Board of Medical Examiners examination (Parts I, II, and III), and residency program directors' ratings. Age and indebtedness at medical school graduation and board certification status were also examined.

Results: Those physicians who stayed in emergency medicine and those who migrated from other specialties into emergency medicine had similar measures of academic performance, but both of these groups had higher academic performance measures and higher board certification rates than did the physicians who moved out of emergency medicine. Those who stayed in emergency medicine had the highest mean debt in the senior year of medical school.

Conclusions: High academic performance and high indebtedness are factors associated with choosing or staying in the specialty of emergency medicine.

Academic Emergency Medicine, 1994, *1*, 443–447. https://onlinelibrary.wiley.com/doi/10.1111/j.1553-2712.1994.tb02524.x

4.2.27   The Changing Healthcare System: A Research Agenda for Medical Education

Gang Xu, Mohammadreza Hojat, J. Jon Veloski, and Joseph S. Gonnella

The volatility in the US healthcare system due to unprecedented changes in its organization, financing, and delivery, coupled with a growing physician surplus in certain areas, suggests the need for a research agenda to investigate the impact of these forces on the educational programs of medical schools. This article discusses the potential impact of trends in the healthcare environment on the following key aspects of undergraduate medical education: admissions, faculty, curriculum, and educational outcomes. A representative set of research questions intended to stimulate inquiry and guide empirical studies in each of the four domains is proposed.

Evaluation and The Health Professions, 1999, 22(2), 152–168.

4.2.28   A National Study of the Factors Influencing Men and Women Physicians' Choices of Primary Care Specialties

Gang Xu, Susan L. Rattner, J. Jon Veloski, Mohammadreza Hojat, Sylvia K. Fields, and Barbara Barzansky

Background: Despite a recent increase in the percentage of graduating US medical students planning to pursue generalist careers, interest in primary care among students is still far below what it was in the early 1980s and falls well short of the stated goal of the Association of American Medical Colleges that half of all graduates should choose generalist careers. Also during the past decade, the number of women students and physicians has increased. Given the importance of concerns regarding the primary care workforce, it is timely to examine the relationship between gender and other factors that influence the decision to enter primary care.

Method: A total of 1038 (65%) men and 558 (35%) women primary care physicians selected from the 1983 and 1984 graduates of all allopathic US medical schools were surveyed in early 1993. Gender comparisons were made on the 19 variables that influenced the physicians' decisions to enter primary care specialties and on the 6 factor scores derived from a factor analysis of these 19 variables. Also included in the gender comparisons were characteristics of practice, populations served, timing of making the decision to enter primary care, and personal demographic information.

Results: Men, more than women, were influenced to become primary care physicians by early role models. Women, more than men, were influenced by personal and family factors. Overall, medical school experience and personal values are two important factors that explained the largest variances of the 19 predictor variables influencing the physicians' choices of primary care disciplines. There was no gender difference in place of origin, family income as a child, timing of the decision to become a primary care physician, or amount of debt upon graduation.

Conclusion: The nationwide study of primary care physicians indicates that men and women physicians differ in their perceptions of the relative importance of factors influencing the choice of a primary care specialty. Gender-specific factors should receive more attention in the development of successful strategies to attract more medical students into primary care specialties.

Academic   Medicine,   1995,   *70*,   398–404.   https://doi.org/10.1097/ACM.0b013e31820bb3e7

4.2.29   A Comparison of Jefferson Medical College Graduates Who Chose Emergency Medicine with Those Who Chose Other Specialties

Gang Xu and J. Jon Veloski

Using the database of the Jefferson Medical College Longitudinal Study of students and graduates, 53 Jefferson graduates who chose emergency medicine (EM) over the decade from 1981 through 1990 were compared with the other Jefferson graduates during that decade who chose other specialties. As seniors, those who chose EM had the highest debt of seniors going into any specialty. However, the mean peak income they expected was higher than expected by the other nonsurgeons, although it was below that expected by the surgeons. The EM group compared favorably with those who chose other specialties in terms of their academic records and had the highest mean Part III score on the National Board of Medical Examiners examination of any of the groups studied. The students who chose EM also indicated their great willingness to see patients from low-income households and were willing to spend more of their practice time serving these groups than the students who chose the other specialties. The authors discuss these findings as related to the nature of EM and medical school graduates' choices of specialties.

Academic   Medicine,   1991,   *66,*   366–368.   https://doi.org/10.1097/ 00001888-199106000-00014

4.2.30   Factors Influencing Physicians' Decisions to Remain in Emergency Medicine

Gang Xu and J. Jon Veloski

Our study examined the factors influencing physicians' decisions to continue their careers in emergency medicine (EM). A questionnaire was sent to 53 graduates (classes of 1981–1990) of Jefferson Medical College whose specialty choices in their senior year had been EM. They were asked to indicate to what extent each of the 23 factors had encouraged them to remain in EM (with 0 = no influence, 1 = minor positive influence, and 4 = major positive influence). Thirty-six physicians (68%) returned usable questionnaires. For the 33 who had remained in EM, the mean scores for the most important factors were as follows: challenging diagnostic problems (3.38); predictable working hours (3.03); intellectual content of the specialty (2.93); income (2.93); and opportunity to deliver primary care (2.91). The mean scores for the least important factors were as follows: examples of family or friends (0.67); minimum patient contact (0.67); fewer malpractice problems (0.83); and encouragement from other physicians (1.16). The level of educational debt was also rated as minor influential factor (1.43).

This study revealed that those who chose EM highly valued the predictable working hours, which reinforces the notion of the importance of lifestyle in influencing physicians' career choice. We previously reported for this same group of physicians that their actual amount of educational indebtedness was highest as compared with the indebtedness of other specialty groups. However, the self-reported data presented here suggest that these physicians' decisions to be emergency doctors were not influenced by indebtedness. This leads us to speculate that physicians might not be consciously aware of the influence of indebtedness on career decisions even though it exists.

Academic   Medicine,   1992,   *67,*   413.   https://doi.org/10.1097/00001888-199206000-00016

4.2.31   Comparing the Academic Performances of Geriatricians and Other Family Physicians and Internists

Gang Xu and J. Jon Veloski

This study compared the academic performances of geriatricians and other family physicians and internists. The sample consisted of the graduates of Jefferson Medical College from 1971 through 1981 whose first board certifications were in either family medicine or internal medicine. Of the family physicians, there were 14 whose second or third certificates were in geriatrics. Of the internists, there were 26 whose second or third certificates were in geriatrics. The graduates who had second or third certificates in areas other than geriatrics were removed from the analysis, leaving 250 family physicians and 197 internists to be compared with the geriatricians in their respective fields.

The graduates who were board certified in family medicine and held geriatrics certificates had better academic performances during medical school than those who were certified only in family medicine. They had significantly ($p < 0.05$) higher freshman and sophomore grade-point averages, clinical clerkship examination scores, and National Board of Medical Examiners (NBME) Part I and Part II examination scores. There was no significant difference between the two groups on the NBME Part III. The academic performances of the graduates who were board certified in internal medicine and held geriatrics certificates were not significantly different from those of the graduates who were certified only in internal medicine. In addition, the academic performances of the geriatricians certified in family medicine were compared with those of the geriatricians certified in internal medicine, showing no significant difference.

Geriatrics is becoming a well-defined field and is one rooted in primary care. This study addresses the public concern about the quality of geriatricians and shows that highly qualified physicians in family medicine and internal medicine are obtaining geriatrics certificates—a positive outcome worthy of investigations in other studies.

Academic   Medicine,   1993,   *68*,   388.   https://doi.org/10.1097/0000
1888-199305000-00027

4.2.32 Comparisons Among Three Types of Generalist Physicians: Personal Characteristics, Medical School Experiences, Financial Aid, and Other Factors Influencing Career Choice

Gang Xu, J. Jon Veloski, Barbara Barzansky, Mohammadreza Hojat, James J. Diamond, and Vincent M. B. Silenzio

A national survey of family physicians, general internists, and general pediatricians was conducted in the USA to examine differences among the three groups of generalist physicians, with particular regard to the factors influencing their choice of generalist career. Family physicians were more likely to have made their career decision before medical school and were more likely to have come from inner-city or rural areas. Personal values and early role models play a very important role in influencing their career choice. In comparison, a higher proportion of general internists had financial aid service obligations, and their choice of the specialty was least influenced by personal values. General pediatricians had more clinical experiences either in primary care or with underserved populations, and they regarded medical school experiences as more important in influencing their specialty choice than did the other two groups. Admission committees may use these specialty-related factors to develop strategies to attract students into each type of generalist career.

Advances in Health Sciences Education, 1996, *1*(3), 197–207.

4.2.33   *Changing Interest in Family Medicine and Students'*
Academic Performance

Gang Xu, J. Jon Veloski, and Mohammadreza Hojat

In recent years, there has been declining interest in family practice among medical school graduates nationwide. Although a change in the proportion of students interested in certain specialties does not necessarily mean a corresponding change in their academic credentials, some recent studies reported a significant decrease in the percentage of top students choosing careers in primary care specialties, including family practice, and a significant increase in the percentage of these top students choosing controllable lifestyle specialties such as anesthesiology, radiology, pathology, and emergency medicine. The study addresses this general question: How do students who choose family medicine compare academically with those who choose other specialties?

The sample consisted of all graduates from Jefferson Medical College from 1980 through 1991 (a total of 12 years). Students' performance in medical school and on the National Board of Medical Examiners (NBME) examinations were collected prospectively as a part of a longitudinal study. Also included in this study was information gathered through a questionnaire given to all seniors before they received the results of the National Resident Matching Program, which included their plans for specialization after the first year of postgraduate training and the community in which they planned to work.

Of the 2263 graduates studied, 385 (17%) preferred family practice, and the proportion decreased from 18.2% in 1980–1982 to 14.7% in 1989–1991. In comparisons of academic performances during medical school, the family medicine group performance was comparable with that of most other specialty groups. Of particular note here were the NBME Part III scores where the family medicine group was ranked the second highest and scored significantly higher than each of the remaining five specialty groups. There was no significant difference in any one of the four measured areas of residency program director ratings among the specialty groups compared. Consistent with national statistics, this study sample demonstrated a decline in the number of students preferring family practice. However, the performance of those in the family medicine group was comparable to that of those in other specialties.

Academic   Medicine,   1993,   *68*(Supplement),   s52–s54.   https://doi. org/10.1097/00001888-199310000-00044

Also in *Proceedings of the Thirty-second Annual Conference on Research in Medical Education*, Washington, DC. November 1993.

4.2.34 Physicians' Intention to Stay in or Leave Primary Care Specialties and Variables Associated with Such Intention

Gang Xu, J. Jon Veloski, Mohammadreza Hojat, and Sylvia K. Fields

A national mail survey of primary care physicians was conducted in 1993 to examine the differences between those who planned to leave and those who planned to stay in primary care disciplines. The physicians who planned to stay in primary care were those who, at the time of choosing primary care specialties, were more influenced by factors such as personal social values, religion, and presence of a role model prior to medical school. Physicians' race, sex, workload, debt, place where they grew up, family income as a child, and timing when they made the decision to enter primary care disciplines are not associated with their plans to stay in or leave primary care disciplines. Findings indicated that personal social values, religious beliefs, and presence of a role model prior to medical school not only influenced physicians' choice of primary care, but also had a lasting effect on their commitment to such choice.

Evaluation and The Health Professions, 1995, *18*, 92–102.
Copyright© 1995. SagePublishing. https://doi.org/10.1177/016327879501800107

4.2.35   Factors Influencing Primary Care Physicians' Choice to Practice in Medically Underserved Areas

Gang Xu, J. Jon Veloski, Mohammadreza Hojat, Robert M. Politzer,
Howard K. Rabinowitz, and Susan L. Rattner

Purpose: To examine the factors associated with primary care physicians' practice location in underserved areas.

Method: The sample was randomly drawn from practicing generalist physicians who graduated in 1983 and 1984 from MD-granting and DO-granting medical schools. The survey was conducted in 1993. A multiple logistic regression model with maximum likelihood procedures was used in which physician's practice location in an underserved area (1 = Yes; 0 = No) was the dependent variable and 15 other variables were used as regressors.

Results: A 75% response rate was obtained. Physicians' underrepresented minority status, the area where the physicians grew up, the interests expressed prior to medical school to care for the underserved, and financial aid obligations were the most significant predictors in the model. The physicians' experiences with primary care or with underserved patients, both during medical school and in residency, were not associated with their decision to locate in an underserved area.

Conclusions: Physician's personal and demographic characteristics are the most important factors influencing decisions to practice in underserved areas. Admission policies that are targeted to applicants with minority backgrounds, who grew up in a rural or inner-city area, and who express a strong interest prior to medical school to practice in the underserved area would likely increase physician manpower in these areas. Supporting the target individuals who have financial obligations is an additional crucial factor.

Academic Medicine, 1997, *72*(October Supplement), S109–S111. https://doi.org/10.1097/00001888-199710001-00037

4.2.36 Factors Influencing Physicians' Choices to Practice in Inner-City or Rural Areas

Gang Xu, J. Jon Veloski, Mohammadreza Hojat, Robert M. Politzer, Howard K. Rabinowitz, and Susan Rattner

In our previously published study of factors influencing physicians' choice to practice in underserved locations, we did not make a distinction between inner-city and rural locations. In this supplementary study, we replicated the previous study by separating out inner-city and rural areas. The findings suggest that the most significant factors in physicians' decision to practice in inner-city locations were the following: expressed interest prior to medical school, being underrepresented minority, and required or elective clinical experiences in primary care. However, the most significant factors in physicians' choices to practice in rural areas were as follows: being a recipient of the National Health Service Corps' financing, interest expressed prior to medical school, gender (being male), and recipient of other financial supports. These findings shed more light on the factors that influence physicians' choices of practice in inner-city and rural locations.

Academic Medicine (Letter to the Editor), 1997, *72*(12), 1026.

This abstract was written by the book editors.

Chapter 5
Psychosocial Attributes

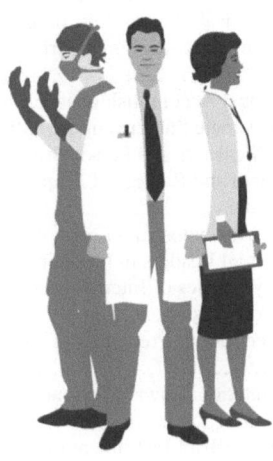

Contents

5.1   Effects of a Brief Curricular Intervention on Medical Students' Attitudes Toward
        People with Disabilities in Healthcare Settings.. 137
5.2   Psychostimulant Drug Abuse and Personality Factors in Medical Students............. 138
5.3   Volunteer Bias in Medical Education Research: An Empirical Study of Over Three
        Decades of Longitudinal Data.. 139
5.4   Economic Diversity in Medical Education: The Relationship Between Students'
        Family Income and Academic Performance, Career Choice, and Student Debt......... 140
5.5   Characteristics of Medical Students Completing an Honors Program in Pathology..... 141
5.6   Biotechnology and Ethics in Medical Education of the New Millennium: Physician
        Roles and Responsibilities.. 142
5.7   Medical Students' Opinions Concerning the Healthcare System......................... 143
5.8   Medical Students' Opinions on Economic Aspects of the Healthcare System.......... 144
5.9   Professional Attitudes and Interpersonal Relationships of Physicians: Are They
        a Problem?... 145
5.10 Perception of Maternal Availability in Childhood and Selected Psychosocial
        Characteristics in Adulthood... 146
5.11 Satisfaction with Early Relationships with Parents and Psychosocial Attributes
        in Adulthood: Which Parent Contributes More?.. 147
5.12 Medical Students' Personal Values and Their Career Choices a Quarter-Century
        Later.. 148
5.13 Students' Personality and Ratings of Clinical Competence in Medical School
        Clerkships: A Longitudinal Study... 149

5.14   Personality Assessments and Outcomes in Medical Education and the Practice
       of Medicine: AMEE Guide No. 79.. 150
5.15   Associations Between Selected Psychosocial Attributes and Ratings of Physician
       Competence... 151
5.16   Physicians' Perceptions of the Changing Healthcare System: Comparisons by
       Gender and Specialties... 152
5.17   Medical Student's Cognitive Appraisal of Stressful Life Events as Related
       to Personality, Physical Well-Being, and Academic Performance: A Longitudinal
       Study.. 153
5.18   Career Satisfaction and Professional Accomplishments................................. 154
5.19   Psychosocial Characteristics of Female Students in the Allied Health and Medical
       Colleges: Psychometrics of the Measures and Personality Profiles..................... 155
5.20   Empathy Scores in Medical School and Ratings of Empathic Behavior
       in Residency Training 3 Years Later... 156
5.21   Can Empathy, Other Personality Attributes, and Level of Positive Social Influence
       in Medical School Identify Potential Leaders in Medicine?............................. 157
5.22   A Comparison of the Personality Profiles of Internal Medicine Residents, Physician
       Role Models, and the General Population.. 158
5.23   Students' Psychosocial Characteristics as Predictors of Academic Performance
       in Medical School.. 159
5.24   Empathic and Sympathetic Orientations Toward Patient Care: Conceptualization,
       Measurement, and Psychometrics.. 160
5.25   Attitudes Toward Managed Care: A Brief Instrument to Measure Attitudes
       of Medical Students Toward Change in the Healthcare System.......................... 161
5.26   Perceptions of Medical School Seniors of the Current Changes in the US
       Healthcare System.. 162
5.27   Underlying Construct of Empathy, Optimism, and Burnout in Medical Students...... 163
5.28   The Devil Is in the Third Year: A Longitudinal Study of Erosion of Empathy
       in Medical School.. 164
5.29   Effects of Academic and Psychosocial Predictors of Performance in Medical
       School on Coefficients of Determination.. 165
5.30   Personality and Specialty Interest in Medical Students................................. 166
5.31   The Relationship Between Grit and Selected Personality Measures in Medical
       Students.. 167
5.32   Predicting Peer Nominations: A Social Network Approach.............................. 168
5.33   Identifying Potential Engaging Leaders Within Medical Education: The Role
       of Positive Influence on Peers... 169
5.34   How Much Do Medical Students Know About Physician Income?........................ 170
5.35   Correlates of Physicians' Endorsement of the Legalization of Physician-Assisted
       Suicide... 171
5.36   Peer Nominations as Related to Academic Attainment, Empathy, Personality,
       and Specialty Interest.. 172
5.37   Intra- and Intercultural Comparisons of Personality Profiles of Medical Students
       in Argentina and the USA.. 173
5.38   Persistent Impostor Phenomenon is Associated with Distress in Medical Students.... 174
5.39   Income Expectations of First-Year Students at Jefferson Medical College
       as a Predictor of Family Practice Specialty Choice..................................... 175
5.40   Mindfulness-Based Stress Reduction Lowers Psychological Distress in Medical
       Students.. 176
5.41   The Income Expectations of Medical Students in the Time Period 1970–1980......... 177
5.42   Students' Certainty During Course Test-Taking and Performance on Clerkships
       and Board Exams... 178

Abstract

- This section includes abstracts of studies on psychosocial attributes in relation to academic performance, clinical competence, specialty interest, and other personal qualities.
- Adding psychosocial measures to predictive performance models significantly improved the magnitude of prediction beyond conventional medical school academic achievement indicators.
- Level of students' certainty of responses to multiple-choice examination questions could identify over- and under-confident students, and using confidence-weighted scoring could improve the psychometrics of examinations.
- Students with lower ratings of clinical competence scored significantly lower on self-esteem and sociability, but higher on loneliness.
- Physicians rated higher on clinical competence scored significantly lower on the anxiety and emotional instability scales, while top-rated physicians reported better relationships with their parents and peers.
- Medical students who reported using psychostimulant drugs compared to nonusers obtained significantly higher scores on a personality measure of aggression-hostility.
- Physicians who at the end of medical school granted permission to researchers to collect performance data on their behalf generally performed better during medical school than others. Women and members of minority groups were less likely to grant permission.
- Students from high-income families performed better in the preclinical phase; however, no significant difference was observed between those from high- and low-income families in the clinical phase of medical school education.
- Empathy erodes in the third year of medical school when curriculum shifts from the preclinical to clinical phase of medical education.
- Psychosocial measures in general and empathic orientation toward patient care in particular were significantly associated with specialty interest.
- Students with high preference for social value were more likely to pursue "people-oriented" over "technology-oriented" specialties, and those with high preference for economic value expected higher peak income after graduation from medical school.
- Internal medicine residents, compared to the general population, were more likely to have deeper intellectual curiosity, higher aspiration, more vivid imagination, and more interest in mental stimulation. Residents, compared to role models in medicine, were less eager to face challenges, less able to control their impulses, and less eager to cope with adversity.
- Hospital-based physicians (anesthesiologists, pathologists, and radiologists) were more likely to endorse legalization of physician-assisted suicide than primary care physicians.
- Career satisfaction was associated with higher satisfaction with medical school education, greater academic and clinical performance, more involvement with teaching and research activities, and higher orientation toward lifelong learning.

- Mindfulness-based stress reduction intervention significantly reduced psychological distress in medical students.
- Medical students reporting that their mothers were unavailable in childhood scored higher on measures of loneliness and depression, and lower on measures of self-esteem and well-being, and appraised stressful events more negatively than others. Those who perceived higher satisfaction with the mother in childhood reported more satisfactory peer relationships.
- Medical students recognized by classmates as the most positive social influencers scored higher on empathy, sociability, activity, and self-esteem, but lower on measures of loneliness, neuroticism, aggression-hostility, and impulsive sensation seeking.
- Those who reported ability to cope better with adversity in life had a more positive personality profile and reported less physical illness.

Keywords Biotechnology and ethics · Burnout · Career satisfaction · Economic diversity · Educational debt · Erosion of empathy · Family income · Grit · Imposter phenomenon · Income expectations · Maternal care · Mindfulness-based stress reduction · Optimism · Peer nomination · Personal values · Personality assessment · Physician-assisted suicide · Positive influencers · Potential leaders · Professional accomplishments · Psychostimulant drugs · Role model · Stressful life events · Student certainty · Volunteer bias

5.1   Effects of a Brief Curricular Intervention on Medical Students' Attitudes Toward People with Disabilities in Healthcare Settings

Paula Bu, J. Jon Veloski, and Nethra S. Ankam

This study sought to evaluate the effects of a brief curricular intervention on medical students' attitudes toward physical disability in healthcare settings. Students participated in a focused curriculum about people with disabilities (PWDs), which included 2.5 h of lectures, panel discussions, and video presentations. After the curricular sessions, students were surveyed ($n = 237$), and their attitudes toward PWDs in healthcare settings were compared with those of students who did not undergo the intervention ($n = 251$) using the Disability Attitudes in Health Care (DAHC) scale. Thematic analysis of the students' comments regarding the session was performed to supplement the DAHC scale. The intervention group responded with significantly more positive attitudes on 6 of the 17 items on the DAHC scale, and multiple linear regression analysis confirmed the independent effect of the curriculum on higher DAHC scale scores. Female students had more positive attitudes on the survey than did male students, although the effect of the curriculum was independent of gender. Previous experiences with PWDs did not correlate to higher attitude scores. These results suggest that a brief curricular intervention on disability can engender more positive attitudes in medical students toward PWDs.

American Journal of Physical Medicine & Rehabilitation, 2016, *95*(12), 939–945. https://journals.lww.com/ajpmr/Fulltext/2016/12000/Effects_of_a_Brief _Curricular_Intervention_on.9.aspx

5.2   Psychostimulant Drug Abuse and Personality Factors in Medical Students

Joshua T. Bucher, Duc M. Vu, and Mohammadreza Hojat

Background: Psychostimulants have a high abuse potential and are appealing to college students for enhancing their examination performance.

Aim: This study was designed to examine the prevalence of psychostimulant drug abuse among medical students and to test the hypothesis that medical students who use psychostimulant drugs for nonmedical reasons are characterized by a sensation-seeking and aggressive-hostility personality and exhibit lower empathy.

Methods: The Zuckerman-Kuhlman personality questionnaire and the Jefferson scale of empathy were completed anonymously online by 321 medical students in 2010–2011 academic year.

Results: A total of 45 students (14%) reported that they had abused psychostimulant medications either before or during medical school. Results of multivariate analysis of variance provided support for one of our research hypotheses: students who reported using psychostimulant compared to the rest obtained a significantly higher average score on the aggressive-hostility personality factor. No other significant differences were observed.

Conclusion: Further research is needed to confirm the rate of psychostimulant drug abusers among medical students in other medical schools. In particular, it is desirable to examine if such psychostimulant drug abusers are likely to abuse other substances in medical school and later in their professional career.

Medical Teacher, 2013, *35*(1), 53–57. https://www.tandfonline.com/doi/full/10.3109/0142159X.2012.731099

5.3   Volunteer Bias in Medical Education Research: An Empirical Study of Over Three Decades of Longitudinal Data

Clara A. Callahan, Mohammadreza Hojat, and Joseph S. Gonnella

Context: The issue of whether medical education research outcomes can be biased by students' refusal to allow their data to be used in outcomes research should be empirically addressed to assure the validity of research findings. Given that institutions are expected to document the outcomes of their educational programs, evaluations of clinical performance subsequent to medical school are crucial, but are often incomplete when graduates decline to permit data collection.

Objectives: This study aimed to examine the demographic and performance differences between research volunteers and others.

Methods: A total of 7415 doctors graduated from Jefferson Medical College between 1970 and 2004; 75% ($n = 5575$) agreed to participate in medical education research by granting written permission for the collection of data from their postgraduate training directors on their behalf (research volunteers); 20% ($n = 1489$) refused to grant such permission (non-volunteers); and 5% ($n = 351$) did not return the permission form (nonrespondents). This prospective longitudinal study compared research volunteers, non-volunteers, and nonrespondents on gender, ethnicity, and performance measures prior to, during, and after medical school, scores on medical licensing examinations, and board certification status.

Results: Doctors who granted permission (volunteers) generally performed better during and after medical school. In addition, they scored higher on medical licensing examinations and had a higher certification rate. Women and members of ethnic minority groups were less likely to grant permission.

Conclusions: The study raises questions about the validity of research findings as a result of volunteerism in medical education research. The implications for guidelines regarding the protection of human subjects in medical education research, and for educational outcomes, are discussed.

Medical Education, 2007, *41*(8), 746–753.   https://onlinelibrary.wiley.com/doi/10.1111/j.1365-2923.2007.02803.x

5.4   Economic Diversity in Medical Education: The Relationship Between Students' Family Income and Academic Performance, Career Choice, and Student Debt

Raelynn Cooter, James B. Erdmann, Joseph S. Gonnella, Clara A. Callahan, Mohammadreza Hojat, and Gang Xu

Providing access to higher education across all income groups is a national priority. This analysis assessed the performance, career choice, and educational indebtedness of medical college students whose educational pursuits were assisted by the provision of financial support. The study looked at designated outcomes (academic performance, specialty choice, accumulated debt) in relation to the independent variable, family (parental) income, of 1464 students who graduated from Jefferson Medical College between 1992 and 2002. Students were classified into groups of high, moderate, and low income based on their parental income. During the basic science years, the high-income group performed better; however, in the clinical years, performance measures were similar. Those in the high-income group tended to pursue surgery, while those in the low-income group preferred family medicine. The mean of accumulated educational debt was significantly higher for the low-income group. The study provides support for maintaining economic diversity in medical education.

Evaluation & The Health Professions, 2004, *27*(3), 252–264.

5.5   Characteristics of Medical Students Completing an Honors Program in Pathology

Bruce A. Fenderson, Mohammadreza Hojat, Ivan Damjanov,
and Emanuel Rubin

The Honors Program in Pathology at Jefferson Medical College provides a voluntary enrichment opportunity for students who have demonstrated a superior ability to cope with the pathology curriculum and who rank in the upper fifth of their class. This study was performed to determine whether honor students possess cognitive and psychosocial attributes that distinguish them from their classmates. Students from five academic years (entering classes 1991–1995) were divided into three groups: (1) those who completed the Honors Program ($n = 85$), (2) those in the top 20% of the class who were offered the option but chose not to participate in the Honors Program ($n = 128$), and (3) those who did not qualify for the program ($n = 953$). Comparisons between these three groups were made on the basis of selected measures of academic achievement retrieved from the Jefferson Longitudinal Study database and psychosocial data obtained from a questionnaire completed during the first-year orientation. Students who completed the Honors Program in Pathology had scored higher on the physical science section of the Medical College Admission Test (MCAT) and had obtained higher first-year grade-point averages than students in both of the other groups. Subsequently, they attained higher second-year grade-point averages and scored higher on Steps 1 and 2 of the United States Medical Licensing Examination (USMLE), compared with their peers in the other groups. There were no significant differences in psychosocial measures between honor students and the rest of the cohort (group 3). However, students in the top 20% of the class who declined the invitation to participate in the Honors Program (group 2) showed higher scores on the Taylor Manifest Anxiety Scale and the Eysenck Emotional Instability (Neuroticism) Scale than their classmates. Despite these differences, students who completed the Honors Program (group 1) and eligible students who declined participation (group 2) selected similar pathways of postgraduate residency training: both groups preferred internal medicine to family practice, and both were more likely than the rest of the cohort to begin residency training at a top-ranked academic/research medical center. Voluntary participation in an Honors Program is a self-selection system that identifies students who are most likely to succeed academically at the highest levels. Residency selection committees may wish to pay close attention to student involvement in similar programs, because this information may provide insights into student personality and general aptitude.

Human Pathology, 1999, *30*(11), 1296–1301.

5.6   Biotechnology and Ethics in Medical Education of the New Millennium: Physician Roles and Responsibilities

Joseph S. Gonnella and Mohammadreza Hojat

Although the medical education curriculum varies internationally, we suggest that it is desirable for medical educators to share a universal responsibility to prepare physicians to perform three distinct yet interrelated professional roles. The first is that of a clinician who has the knowledge and technical skills to care for individual patients as well as the public. The second role can be viewed as that of an educator, a teacher, or a consultant who has the interpersonal skills and personal qualities to teach, advise, and counsel patients and the public about their health and illness, risk factors, and healthy lifestyle. The third role is that of a resource manager to enable physicians to care for patients and serve the public not only by drawing on available material assets but also by prudent use of the resources for better serving the most number of people at the least expense without compromising the quality of care. The very nature of the medical profession also obligates medical educators throughout the world to sensitize medical students and physicians to the ethical responsibilities that are implicit to each of the three aforementioned roles. Although the basic ethical responsibilities of do no harm and confidentiality are universal, certain global changes, such as rapid advancements in biotechnology and resource allocation, are now reshaping medical ethics on every continent. Spawned by the rapid advances in the biomedical sciences, biotechnology is revolutionizing human reproduction, sustaining human life, cloning human beings, and mapping the entire human genetic terrain. These advances imply changes in medical education and the formal preparation of physicians in performing their roles as clinicians, educators, and resource managers. These biotechnological developments, coupled with the increasing cost of health care and maldistribution of resources worldwide, present unprecedented ethical-social challenges that need to be addressed in the education of the physician in the new millennium.

Medical Teacher, 2001, *23*(4), 371–377. https://www.tandfonline.com/doi/abs/ 10.1080/01421590120042982

5.7   Medical Students' Opinions Concerning the Healthcare System

Mary W. Herman

The opinions of freshman and senior medical students on major health system problems and policies were investigated in 1980–1981. Responses of 214 freshmen and 203 seniors are reported in four major areas: (1) physician dominance of the healthcare system, (2) autonomy in patient care, (3) availability of services, and (4) preventive and social aspects of care. With respect to physician dominance, more seniors (63%) than freshman (44%) agree that physicians should determine health policy and that dominance over other health personnel is necessary (75% and 61%, respectively). Professional review of patient care is generally acceptable to both classes, but more freshmen than seniors agree that evaluation should be a condition for relicensure. Less than a fifth of the students in either class believe that patients should be told as little as possible or that they should accept the authority of doctors without question. More freshmen than seniors consider the availability of medical care as a major problem (76% and 58%, respectively), and similar proportions believe that it is the responsibility of the government to assure access to all. Freshmen and seniors generally agree on the need for greater emphasis on prevention and social aspects of illness. Because of the important role played by physicians in the healthcare system, it is recommended that serious attention be devoted to education in this area, even though it may have a limited impact on professional attitudes.

Journal of Community Health, 1984, *9*(3), 196–205. https://pubmed.ncbi.nlm.nih.gov/6480887/

5.8   Medical Students' Opinions on Economic Aspects
of the Healthcare System

Mary W. Herman

Responses of 423 freshmen and 410 seniors at Jefferson Medical College in 1980–1981 and 1982–1983 to 15 questions on economic aspects of the healthcare system were compared. A majority of students considered the cost of medical care, cost of medical education, malpractice claims, and failure of individuals to assume responsibility for their health to be major problems. A majority of seniors also considered excessive government influence on the financing of medical care as a major problem. More freshmen than seniors favored national health insurance and health maintenance organizations. More seniors than freshmen supported the professional standards review organization concept and action to discourage increases in the supply of physicians. Concern about the number of physicians entering the profession increased among seniors between 1981 and 1983. The data suggest that at graduation the students were more concerned about the position of physicians but might not be more informed about important aspects of the functioning of the healthcare system than they were at entry.

Journal of Medical Education, 1985, *60*, 431–438. https://doi.org/10.1097/00001888-198506000-00001

Also in *Proceedings of the Twenty-Third Annual Conference on Research in Medical Education*, Chicago, IL, October 1984; 329–334.

5.9   Professional Attitudes and Interpersonal Relationships of Physicians: Are They a Problem?

Mary W. Herman, J. Jon Veloski, and Mohammadreza Hojat

The study used the ratings of recent graduates from Jefferson Medical College to address two questions of major importance to medical educators: (1) How extensive is the problem of poor professional attitudes? (2) Are low ratings on professional attitudes associated with low ratings in other areas of competence? The study sample comprised of 496 individuals who graduated in the years 1978 through 1980. Ratings were obtained from hospitals in which the graduates took their first year of postgraduate training. Fewer than 5% of the graduates received the lowest possible rating on any item, and the majority of the 5% received the lowest rating on ability to handle anxiety-producing situations, admit to an error in judgment, devote sufficient time to their work, seek help when needed, and relate to other healthcare personnel. The ratings were then related to whether or not the rating institution would offer the resident further training. Ninety percent of the sample would be made such an offer. Only those graduates with low ratings in all four noncognitive areas were likely not to be offered further residency training. Ratings on professional attitudes were more closely related to the residency offers than were the ratings on knowledge or data gathering skills, but ratings on clinical judgment were more important than professional attitudes. The study supports the view that there is a problem of poor professional attitudes among physicians, and this problem is not always associated with poor performance in other areas. It can be concluded that, despite the difficulties involved in evaluating clinical competence, regularly obtained ratings from a number of observers can provide adequate information on remedial action, and it is important that medical schools assume this responsibility.

Proceedings of the Twenty-First Annual Conference on Research in Medical Education, Washington, DC. 1982, 117–120.
This abstract was written by the book editors.

5.10   Perception of Maternal Availability in Childhood and Selected Psychosocial Characteristics in Adulthood

Mohammadreza Hojat

The associations between reported perception of maternal availability in childhood and a set of psychosocial measures in adulthood were examined. Participants were 362 medical students who were divided into three groups based on their retrospective report of maternal availability before their fifth birthday: mothers mostly available ($n = 260$), partly available ($n = 70$), and mostly unavailable ($n = 32$). Those with mostly unavailable mothers scored significantly higher on the intensity and chronicity of loneliness scales, reported more depression, scored lower on self-esteem, perceived themselves as less healthy, evaluated the same stressful events more negatively, and perceived both of their parents more negatively than those with mostly available mothers.

Genetic, Social, and General Psychology Monographs, 1996, *122*, 425–450. https://pubmed.ncbi.nlm.nih.gov/8976598/

5.11 Satisfaction with Early Relationships with Parents and Psychosocial Attributes in Adulthood: Which Parent Contributes More?

Mohammadreza Hojat

The relationships between perceived satisfaction with early relationships with parents and adults' psychosocial attributes were addressed in this study. The participants were 928 medical students (37% women) who completed a set of personality questionnaires. The results indicated that perceived satisfaction with the mother in childhood was significantly associated with less intensity and chronicity of loneliness, less depression, less anxiety, a less negative view of stressful life events, higher self-esteem, and more satisfaction with peer relationships. No significant association was found between perceived satisfaction with the father and these personality measures. The results are discussed in the context of attachment theory and internal working models.

Journal of Genetic Psychology, 1998, *159*, 203–220. https://www.tandfonline.com/doi/abs/10.1080/00221329809596146

5.12 Medical Students' Personal Values and Their Career Choices a Quarter-Century Later

Mohammadreza Hojat, Timothy P. Brigham, Edward Gottheil, Gang Xu, Karen Glaser, and J. Jon Veloski

A longitudinal study of 391 physicians tested two hypotheses regarding personal values and career choices: that higher preference for social values would be associated with physicians' being more interested in "people-oriented" rather than "technology-oriented" specialties and that higher preference for economic values would be associated with expectations of high income. The physicians (344 men, 47 women) were graduates of Jefferson Medical College in 1974 and 1975 who completed the Allport-Vernon-Lindzey Study of Values during medical school. Analysis showed that physicians currently in the "people-oriented" specialties scored significantly higher on the social value scale than their peers in "technology-oriented" specialties. A moderate but statistically significant correlation was found between scores on the economic value scale and expectations of higher income. The findings suggest that physicians' personal values are relevant to their career decisions such as specialty choice and expectations of income. The findings have implications with regard to two major issues in the evolving healthcare system, namely, the distribution of physicians by specialty and cost containment.

Psychological Reports, 1998, *83*, 243–248.

Copyright© 1998. Sage Publishing. https://journals.sagepub.com/doi/pdf/10.2466/pr0.1998.83.1.243

5.13   Students' Personality and Ratings of Clinical Competence in Medical School Clerkships: A Longitudinal Study

Mohammadreza Hojat, Clara A. Callahan, and Joseph S. Gonnella

This study was designed to examine the associations between students' personality and assessments of their clinical competence in medical school. A set of questionnaires were completed by 1710 medical students to measure their self-esteem, sociability, loneliness, general anxiety, test anxiety, neuroticism (emotionality), perceptions of early relationships with parents, and general health. Students were divided into three groups of the low, moderate, and high competent based on the number of "honors" ratings they received in core clinical clerkships during their third year of medical school. Multivariate statistical analyses showed that the low competent students scored significantly lower on the self-esteem and sociability, but higher on the loneliness scale. The low competent students also perceived their early relationships with their parents as less satisfactory. Findings suggest that medical students' clinical competence assessments are associated with some aspects of their personality and with perceptions of early relationships with their parents. Findings have implications for the development of educational remedies and counseling strategies.

Psychology, Health & Medicine, 2004, *9*(2), 247–252. https://www.tandfonline.com/doi/full/10.1080/13548500410001670771

5.14   Personality Assessments and Outcomes in Medical Education and the Practice of Medicine: AMEE Guide No. 79

Mohammadreza Hojat, James B. Erdmann, and Joseph S. Gonnella

In a paradigm of physician performance we propose that both "cognitive" and "noncognitive" components contribute to the performance of physicians in training and in practice. Our review of the relevant literature indicates that personality, as an important factor of the "noncognitive" component, plays a significant role in academic and professional performances. We describe findings on 14 selected personality instruments in predicting academic and professional performances. We question the contention that personality can be validly and reliably assessed from admission interviews, letters of recommendation, essays, and personal statements. Based on the conceptual relevance and currently available empirical evidence, we propose that personality attributes such as conscientiousness and empathy should be considered among the measures of choice for the assessment of pertinent aspects of personality in academic and professional performance. Further exploration is needed to search for additional personality attributes pertinent to medical education and patient care. Implications for career counseling, assessments of professional development and medical education outcomes, and potential use as supplementary information for admission decisions are discussed.

Hojat, M., Erdmann, J.B., & Gonnella, J.S. (2014). AMEE Guide 79: Personality assessments and outcomes in medical education and the practice of medicine. Dundee, UK: *Association for Medical Education in Europe (AMEE)*.

Reprinted as an independent book from the following invited article: *Medical Teacher*, 2014, *35*(7) e1267–e1301. https://www.tandfonline.com/doi/full/10.3109/0142159X.2013.785654

5.15 Associations Between Selected Psychosocial Attributes and Ratings of Physician Competence

Mohammadreza Hojat, Karen M. Glaser, and J. Jon Veloski

Objective: To investigate the associations between selected psychosocial attributes and ratings of clinical competence of physicians.

Methods: Participants were 110 physicians (52% of the total class who graduated from the Jefferson Medical College of Thomas Jefferson University in 1991 [38% women]). They completed the psychosocial questionnaires voluntarily while in medical school and also granted written permission to collect clinical competence ratings from their residency program directors.

Psychosocial Measures: Included Taylor Manifest Anxiety Scale, Emotional Instability, Extraversion, Rosenberg Self-Esteem Scale, UCLA Loneliness, Beck Depression Inventory, measures of poor relationships, and satisfaction with early relationships with mothers and fathers.

Outcome Measures: Included physician clinical competence ratings in three areas of clinical competence: data gathering skills, interpersonal relations and attitudes, and socioeconomic aspects of patient care.

Results: Results showed that physicians rated in the top half in any clinical competence area scored significantly lower on the anxiety and emotional instability scales than their counterparts in the bottom half of the clinical competence measures. Also, top-rated physicians reported better peer relationships than their bottom-rated counterparts. With regard to the perceptions of early relationships with parents, perceptions of warm relationships with fathers in childhood were not significantly associated with clinical competence ratings, but physicians in the top half of the rating distribution of interpersonal relations and attitudes and socioeconomic aspects of patient care reported warmer relationships with their mothers than their counterparts in the bottom half of the distributions.

Academic Medicine, 1996, *71*(Supplement), S103–S105. https://doi.org/10.1097/00001888-199610000-00059

5.16   Physicians' Perceptions of the Changing Healthcare System: Comparisons by Gender and Specialties

Mohammadreza Hojat, Joseph S. Gonnella, James B. Erdmann, J. Jon Veloski, Daniel Z. Louis, Thomas J. Nasca, and Susan L. Rattner

This study was designed to investigate physicians' perceptions of changes in the US healthcare system impacting academic medicine, quality of care, patient referrals, cost, and ethical and sociopolitical aspects of medicine. A survey was mailed in 1998 to 1272 physicians (graduates of Jefferson Medical College between 1987 and 1992); 835 physicians (66%) responded. Results showed that substantial majority (92%) believed that learning to work in a managed care environment should become an essential component of medical education. Physicians perceived that current changes impair physicians' autonomy (94%) and restrain physician's freedom to provide optimal care (84%). A sizable majority (75%) endorsed patients' freedom to seek specialist care, and 55% believed that capitation reduces physicians' motivation for long-term monitoring of patients. The majority endorsed universal health coverage (80%) and agreed to support rather than resist the changes (62%). Only 18% hold a positive view of the changes in the future. The majority believed that medical education should prepare physicians to provide end-of-life care (92%) and that organized medicine should take a stand on social issues that can influence the well-being of society (79%). Only 34% endorsed the legalization of physician-assisted suicide. No gender differences were observed, but a few differences were found between generalists and specialists. Results can help in understanding physicians' perceptions of current changes in the United States.

Journal of Community Health, 2000, 25(6), 455–471. https://link.springer.com/article/10.1023/A:1005192613992

5.17   Medical Student's Cognitive Appraisal of Stressful Life Events as Related to Personality, Physical Well-Being, and Academic Performance: A Longitudinal Study

Mohammadreza Hojat, Joseph S. Gonnella, James B. Erdmann, and Wolfgang H. Vogel

This longitudinal study was designed to test three hypotheses that medical students who can cope better with adversity would (1) have a more positive personality profile, (2) report less physical illnesses, and (3) perform better academically. Total participants were 2114 medical students at Jefferson Medical College who completed a set of psychosocial questionnaires and were prospectively followed up during medical school education and beyond. Participants reported on a five-point scale their appraisal of five stressors (death or health deterioration of a family member, personal illness, financial and academic problems). Students who experienced the stressors ($n = 1446$, 68% of total participants) were divided into three groups (resilient, intermediate, frail) based on their appraisal of the stressors. The three groups were compared on a set of personality scales (e.g., general anxiety, depression, test anxiety, neuroticism, loneliness, self-esteem, and extraversion), physical well-being factors (e.g., chronic health, eating/drinking/smoking, agitation symptoms, somatic symptoms, and global sickness), academic performance indicators in medical school (e.g., grade-point averages, class rank, and medical licensing examinations), and ratings of clinical competence in postgraduate medical training. Hypotheses 1 and 2 were confirmed, and hypothesis 3 was partially confirmed. Implications for developing coping skills, stress management strategies, and student counseling are discussed.

Personality and Individual Differences, 2003, *35*(1), 219–235.

5.18   Career Satisfaction and Professional Accomplishments

Mohammadreza Hojat, Benjamin Kowitt, Cataldo Doria,
and Joseph S. Gonnella

Context: Research on doctor career satisfaction has often focused on factors such as income, specialty, gender, work hours, autonomy, patient load, lifestyle preferences, work environment, and insurance regulations. Other educational, personal, and professional factors have not received sufficient empirical attention.

Objective: This study was designed to test the following five hypotheses that doctors' career satisfaction is associated with: (1) higher satisfaction with their undergraduate medical education; (2) greater academic and clinical competence; (3) more involvement in teaching and research activities; (4) higher orientation toward lifelong learning; and (5) increased professional accomplishments.

Methods: A survey was mailed in 2006 to a national sample of 5349 doctors in the USA who graduated from Jefferson Medical College between 1975 and 2000; 3170 (59%) returned completed surveys. Based on responses to a career satisfaction question, doctors were classified into three groups: highly satisfied (top third, $n = 1078$); moderately satisfied (middle third, $n = 1031$); and least satisfied (bottom third, $n = 1061$). These groups were compared on a number of variables.

Results: All five research hypotheses were confirmed. Additionally, no significant association was observed between career satisfaction, age, years in practice, gender, or ethnicity; however, career satisfaction was associated with doctors' specialties.

Conclusions: The findings suggest that factors such as satisfaction with medical education; medical school class rank; assessments of clinical competence, teaching, and research activities; orientation toward lifelong learning; and professional accomplishments should be considered for a more comprehensive understanding of doctors' career satisfaction.

Medical Education, 2010, *44*(10), 969–976. https://onlinelibrary.wiley.com/doi/10.1111/j.1365-2923.2010.03735.x

5.19   Psychosocial Characteristics of Female Students in the Allied Health and Medical Colleges: Psychometrics of the Measures and Personality Profiles

Mohammadreza Hojat and Kevin Lyons

For the purpose of developing a comprehensive assessment method of predicting academic and professional success among health professions students, a set of 12 psychosocial measures were administered, and their psychometric properties were examined. Participants were 141 female allied health and 71 female medical students. Alpha and test-retest reliabilities and construct and concurrent validities of the measures were studied, and most of the measures were found to have satisfactory psychometric properties. Comparisons were also made between medical and allied health sciences students using the 12 psychosocial measures. Allied health students scored higher on loneliness, anxiety, and depression and scored lower on perception of general health and perception of their fathers as compared to medical students. Implications of the findings for development of prediction models of academic and professional performance are discussed.

Advances in Health Sciences Education, 1998, *3*(2), 119–132.

5.20   Empathy Scores in Medical School and Ratings of Empathic Behavior in Residency Training 3 Years Later

Mohammadreza Hojat, Salvatore Mangione, Thomas J. Nasca,
Joseph S. Gonnella, and Mike Magee

The authors designed the present study to examine the association between individuals' scores on the Jefferson Scale of Physician Empathy, a self-report empathy scale, during medical school and ratings of their empathic behavior made by directors of their residency training programs 3 years later. Participants were 106 physicians. The authors examined the relationships between scores on the JSPE (with 20 Likert-type items) at the beginning of the students' third year of medical school and ratings of their empathic behavior made by directors of their residency training programs. Top scorers on the JSPE in medical school, compared to bottom scorers, obtained a significantly higher average rating of empathic behavior in residency 3 years later ($p < 0.05$, effect size = 0.50). The findings support the long-term predictive validity of the self-report empathy scale, JSPE, despite different methods of evaluations (self-report and supervisors' ratings) and despite a time interval between evaluations (3 years). Because empathy is relevant to prosocial and helping behavior, it is important for investigators to further enhance our understanding of its correlates and outcomes among health professionals.

The Journal of Social Psychology, 2005, *145*(6), 663–672. https://www.tandfonline.com/doi/abs/10.3200/SOCP.145.6.663-672

5.21   Can Empathy, Other Personality Attributes, and Level of Positive Social Influence in Medical School Identify Potential Leaders in Medicine?

Mohammadreza Hojat, Barret Michalec, J. Jon Veloski, and Mark L. Tykocinski

Purpose: To test the hypotheses that medical students recognized by peers as the most positive social influencers would score (1) high on measures of engaging personality attributes that are conducive to relationship building (empathy, sociability, activity, self-esteem) and (2) low on disengaging personality attributes that are detrimental to interpersonal relationships (loneliness, neuroticism, aggression-hostility, impulsive sensation seeking).

Method: The study sample included 666 Jefferson Medical College students who graduated in 2011–2013. Students used a peer nomination instrument to identify classmates who had a positive influence on their professional and personal development. At matriculation, these students had completed a survey that included the Jefferson Scale of Empathy and Zuckerman-Kuhlman Personality Questionnaire short form and abridged versions of the Rosenberg Self-Esteem Scale and the UCLA Loneliness Scale. In multivariate analyses of variance, the method of contrasted groups was used to compare the personality attributes of students nominated most frequently by their peers as positive influencers (top influencers [top 25% in their class distribution], $n = 176$) with those of students nominated least frequently (bottom influencers [bottom 25%], $n = 171$).

Results: The top influencers scored significantly higher on empathy, sociability, and activity and significantly lower on loneliness compared with the bottom influencers. However, the effect size estimates of the differences were moderate at best.

Conclusions: The research hypotheses were partially confirmed. Positive social influencers appear to possess personality attributes conducive to relationship building, which is an important feature of effective leadership. The findings have implications for identifying and training potential leaders in medicine.

Academic   Medicine,   2015,   *90*,   505–510.   https://doi.org/10.1097/ ACM.0000000000000652

5.22   A Comparison of the Personality Profiles of Internal Medicine Residents, Physician Role Models, and the General Population

Mohammadreza Hojat, Thomas J. Nasca, Mike Magee, Kendra Feeney, Rudolfo Pascual, Frank Urbano, and Joseph S. Gonnella

Purpose: To compare personality profiles of internal medicine residents with those of the general population and positive role models in medicine.

Method: A widely used personality inventory, NEO PI-R(c), which measures 5 major personality factors and 30 important personality facets, was administered to 104 physicians in internal medicine residency and to a nationwide sample of 188 physicians selected as positive role models in medicine.

Results: The internal medicine residents, compared with the general population, were more likely to be attentive, to have deeper intellectual curiosity, to have higher aspiration levels, to have more vivid imagination, to be more receptive to their emotions, to be interested in mental stimulation, and to think carefully before acting. The residents, compared with role models in medicine, were less eager to face challenges, less able to control their impulses, less able to cope with adversity, less easygoing, and less relaxed, but were more likely to crave excitement.

Conclusion: Internal medicine residents and positive role models in medicine have some distinct personal qualities. Understanding the qualities of successful physicians can be helpful in career counseling of medical students and young physicians.

Academic   Medicine,   1999,   *74*,   54–60.   https://doi.org/10.1097/0000 1888-199912000-00017

5.23 Students' Psychosocial Characteristics as Predictors of Academic Performance in Medical School

Mohammadreza Hojat, Mary R. Robeson, Ivan Damjanov, J. Jon Veloski, Karen Glaser, and Joseph S. Gonnella

This study was designed to investigate the incremental effects of selected psychosocial measures—beyond the effects of conventional admission measures—in predicting students' academic performances in medical school. In 1989–1990, 210 second-year students at Jefferson Medical College were each asked to complete 11 psychosocial questionnaires that were then used as predictors of performance measures in medical school. The students' scores on three subtests of the Medical College Admission Test (MCAT) were also used as predictors. Three composite measures of performance were used as the criterion measures: basic science examination grades, clinical examination grades, and ratings of clinical competence. A multiple regression algorithm (general linear model) was used for statistical analysis. The response rate was 83% (175 students). When the psychosocial measures were added to the statistical models in which the common variances of the MCAT scores were already determined, significant increments in the common variances were observed for two of the three performance measures: basic science grades and clinical examination grades. Whereas only 4% of the common variance in the ratings of clinical competence could be accounted for by the MCAT scores, 14% could be accounted for by the psychosocial measures.

The "noncognitive," or psychosocial, measures increased the magnitude of the relationships between the predictive and criterion measures of the students' academic performances beyond the magnitude attained when only the conventional measures should be considered as significant and unique predictors of performance in medical school.

Academic Medicine, 1993, *68*, 635–637. https://doi.org/10.1097/00001888-199308000-00015

5.24   Empathic and Sympathetic Orientations Toward Patient Care: Conceptualization, Measurement, and Psychometrics

Mohammadreza Hojat, John Spandorfer, Daniel Z. Louis, and Joseph S. Gonnella

Purpose: To develop instruments for measuring empathic and sympathetic orientations in patient care and to provide evidence in support of their psychometrics.

Method: Third-year medical students at Jefferson Medical College responded to four clinical vignettes in 2010. For each vignette, students indicated the extent of their agreement with an empathic response (conveying their understanding of patients' concerns) and with a sympathetic response (sharing patients' feelings). The authors calculated, based on students' responses to the clinical vignettes, two measures of empathic and sympathetic orientation. Students also completed the Jefferson Scale of Empathy (JSE) and the Interpersonal Reactivity Index (IRI).

Results: Of the 258 students in the class, 201 (78%) responded to all four vignettes and completed the JSE and IRI. The authors confirmed construct validity of the measures of empathic and sympathetic orientation through factor analysis. The empathic orientation was significantly associated with the measure of empathy (as measured by the JSE) but not with measures of sympathy (as measured by specific scales of the IRI). Conversely, sympathetic orientation was significantly associated with measures of sympathy. Thus, these results support the validity of the empathic and sympathetic orientation measures as assessed by four clinical vignettes. Coefficient alphas for the two measures were, respectively, 0.79 and 0.84.

Conclusions: The validated measures of empathic and sympathetic orientation provide research opportunities to enhance the understanding of the contributions of empathy and sympathy to physicians' competence and patient outcomes.

Academic   Medicine,   2011,   *86*(8),   989–995.   https://doi.org/10.1097/ACM.0b013e31822203d8

5.25   Attitudes Toward Managed Care: A Brief Instrument to Measure Attitudes of Medical Students Toward Change in the Healthcare System

Mohammadreza Hojat, J. Jon Veloski, Joseph S. Gonnella, James B. Erdmann, and Susan L. Rattner

Background: Efforts are being made to prepare medical students, residents, practicing physicians, and medical educators to face new challenges in the evolving healthcare systems. In this critical period of development, it is timely and important to understand the attitudes of medical students toward the changes and their perceived impacts. This study was designed to develop a research instrument to measure medical students' attitudes toward changes in the US healthcare system.

Methods: Based on the literature review, a preliminary draft of a questionnaire (40-item) was developed. After a pilot study the questionnaire was modified and a new version was administered to 394 medical school seniors in 1997 and 1998.

Results: Correlational analyses including factor analysis resulted in a brief attitude scale (8-item) with satisfactory psychometric properties. Data support the face validity, construct validity, criterion-related validity, and alpha reliability of the scale.

Conclusions: This psychometrically sound research instrument can be used in the assessment of educational programs to improve medical students' attitudes toward changes in the healthcare system. Further research is needed to expand this research tool for assessing physicians' attitudes toward different aspects of changes in the US healthcare system.

Academic Medicine, 1999, *74*(October Supplement), S78–S80. https://doi.org/10.1097/00001888-199910000-00046

5.26   Perceptions of Medical School Seniors of the Current Changes in the US Healthcare System

Mohammadreza Hojat, J. Jon Veloski, Daniel Z. Louis, Gang Xu, David Ibarra, Jonathan E. Gottlieb, and James B. Erdmann

Perceptions of medical school seniors about changes occurring in the healthcare environment were investigated. A survey was completed by 196 Jefferson Medical College seniors in the class of 1997. Of the respondents, 79% believed that cost reduction rather than quality of care is the primary consideration behind recent changes, 78% felt that managed care organizations hamper physicians' abilities to render optimal care, 83% maintained that the control of health care by insurance companies would lead to lower quality of care, 69% agreed that patients should have the freedom to seek a specialist's care without being referred by a primary care physician, 82% recommended that mentally ill patients should be referred to a mental health professional, and 82% believed that learning to work in a managed care environment should be an essential component of medical education. Assessment of student perceptions can assist in the development and implementation of appropriate curricular changes.

Evaluation & The Health Professions, 1999, 22(2), 169–183.

5.27   Underlying Construct of Empathy, Optimism, and Burnout in Medical Students

Mohammadreza Hojat, Michael Vergare, Gerald Isenberg, Mitchell Cohen, and John Spandorfer

Objectives: This study was designed to explore the underlying construct of measures of empathy, optimism, and burnout in medical students.

Methods: Three instruments for measuring empathy (Jefferson Scale of Empathy, JSE), optimism (the Life Orientation Test-Revised, LOT-R), and burnout (the Maslach Burnout Inventory, MBI, which includes three scales of emotional exhaustion, depersonalization, and personal accomplishment) were administered to 265 third-year students at Sidney Kimmel (formerly Jefferson) Medical College at Thomas Jefferson University. Data were subjected to factor analysis to examine relationships among measures of empathy, optimism, and burnout in a multivariate statistical model.

Results: Factor analysis (principal component with oblique rotation) resulted in two underlying constructs, each with an eigenvalue greater than one. The first factor involved "positive personality attributes" (factor coefficients greater than 0.58 for measures of empathy, optimism, and personal accomplishment). The second factor involved "negative personality attributes" (factor coefficients greater than 0.78 for measures of emotional exhaustion and depersonalization).

Conclusions: Results confirmed that an association exists between empathy in the context of patient care and personality characteristics that are conducive to relationship building, and considered to be "positive personality attributes," as opposed to personality characteristics that are considered as "negative personality attributes" that are detrimental to interpersonal relationships. Implications for the professional development of physicians in training and in practice are discussed.

International Journal of Medical Education, 2015, 6, 12–16. https://doi.org/10.5116/ijme.54c3.60cd

5.28   The Devil Is in the Third Year: A Longitudinal Study of Erosion of Empathy in Medical School

Mohammadreza Hojat, Michael Vergare, Kaye Maxwell, George Brainard, Steven K. Herrine, Gerald A. Isenberg, J. Jon Veloski, and Joseph S. Gonnella

Purpose: This longitudinal study was designed to examine changes in medical students' empathy during medical school and to determine when the most significant changes occur.

Method: Four hundred fifty-six students who entered Jefferson Medical College in 2002 ($n = 227$) and 2004 ($n = 229$) completed the Jefferson Scale of Physician Empathy at five different times: at entry into medical school on orientation day and subsequently at the end of each academic year. Statistical analyses were performed for the entire cohort, as well as for the "matched" cohort (participants who identified themselves at all five test administrations) and the "unmatched" cohort (participants who did not identify themselves in all five test administrations).

Results: Statistical analyses showed that empathy scores did not change significantly during the first 2 years of medical school. However, a significant decline in empathy scores was observed at the end of the third year which persisted until graduation. Findings were similar for the matched cohort ($n = 121$) and for the rest of the sample (unmatched cohort, $n = 335$). Patterns of decline in empathy scores were similar for men and women and across specialties.

Conclusions: It is concluded that a significant decline in empathy occurs during the third year of medical school. It is ironic that the erosion of empathy occurs during a time when the curriculum is shifting toward patient care activities; this is when empathy is most essential. Implications for retaining and enhancing empathy are discussed.

Academic   Medicine,   2009,   *84*(9),   1182–1191.   https://doi.org/10.1097/ACM.0b013e3181b17e55

5.29   Effects of Academic and Psychosocial Predictors of Performance in Medical School on Coefficients of Determination

Mohammadreza Hojat, Wolfgang H. Vogel, Carter Zeleznik, and Bette D. Borenstein

This study was designed to answer the following questions: (1) Does a set of selected noncognitive variables predict medical school performance measures? (2) Is there a significant increase in the coefficients of determination when noncognitive measures are added to the conventional cognitive predictors in regression models? Complete data on all measures were available for 88 sophomore medical students. Cognitive (academic) predictors were undergraduate GPA in science and non-science courses and scores on science problems, reading, and quantitative scales of the Medical College Admission Test. Noncognitive (psychological) predictors were scores on scales of stressful life events; general anxiety; test anxiety; emotionality; external locus of control; intensity and chronicity of loneliness; sociability; self-esteem; perception of early relationships with mother, father, and peers; and indices of over- and under-confidence. Criterion measures were freshman and sophomore GPAs in medical school and scores on Part I of the National Board Examinations. Results indicate that (1) noncognitive predictors could significantly predict criterion measures and (2) inclusion of noncognitive measures in a model of cognitive predictors could substantially increase the magnitude of the relationships.

Psychological Reports, 1988, *63*, 383–394.
  https://journals.sagepub.com/doi/abs/10.2466/pr0.1988.63.2.383

5.30   Personality and Specialty Interest in Medical Students

Mohammadreza Hojat and Marvin Zuckerman

Background: Research on the relationship between personality and specialty interest is important because of its implications in student career counseling and in forecasting future specialty distribution.

Aim: This study was designed to test the following hypotheses: (1) Students interested in "surgical" specialties would obtain higher scores on a measure of "impulsive sensation seeking" and lower scores on a measure of "neuroticism-anxiety." (2) Students interested in "hospital-based" specialties would score lower on a measure of "sociability" whereas those interested in "primary care" would score higher on this measure. In addition to these two hypotheses, gender differences on personality were also examined.

Method: Study participants were 1076 students who matriculated at Jefferson Medical College between 2002 and 2006. A short version of the Zuckerman-Kuhlman personality questionnaire (ZKPQ) measuring five personality factors of "impulsive sensation seeking," "neuroticism-anxiety," "aggression-hostility," "sociability," and "activity" was completed by research participants at the beginning of medical school. Students were also asked to note their specialty interests.

Results: Multivariate statistical analyses confirmed the first and partially confirmed the second research hypotheses. Results also showed that men scored higher on "impulsive sensation seeking," and women outscored men in the "neuroticism-anxiety" and "activity" scales.

Conclusions: Findings suggest that information about the personalities of medical students can help to predict their career interests. Implications for career counseling are discussed.

Medical Teacher, 2008, *30*, 400–406.   https://www.tandfonline.com/doi/full/10.1080/01421590802043835

5.31   The Relationship Between Grit and Selected Personality Measures in Medical Students

Gerald Isenberg, Andrew M. Brown, Jennifer DeSantis, J. Jon Veloski,
and Mohammadreza Hojat

Objectives: To test the hypothesis that scores on a grit scale are positively associated with personality measures that are conducive to relationship building (empathy, self-esteem, activity, and sociability), but inversely associated with personality measures that are detrimental to interpersonal relationships (neuroticism-anxiety, aggression-hostility, impulsive sensation seeking, and loneliness).

Methods: Convenient sampling was used that included 241 medical students at Sidney Kimmel Medical College at Thomas Jefferson University who participated in this ex post facto research. Validated instruments were used to measure grit, empathy, self-esteem, activity, sociability, neuroticism-anxiety, aggression-hostility, impulsive sensation seeking, and loneliness. Bivariate correlations and multivariate regression were used to examine relationships between scores on the grit scale and personality measures.

Results: Results of bivariate correlational analyses showed that scores on the grit scale were positively and significantly ($p < 0.01$) correlated with measures of self-esteem ($r = 0.35$), empathy ($r = 0.26$), and activity ($r = 0.17$), but negatively and significantly ($p < 0.01$) correlated with measures of loneliness ($r = -0.28$), aggression-hostility ($r = -0.23$), neuroticism-anxiety ($r = -0.22$), and impulsive sensation seeking ($r = -0.18$). Regression analysis indicated that in a multivariate model, higher scores on self-esteem and empathy and lower scores on aggression-hostility were uniquely and significantly associated with grit scores ($R = 0.43, p < 0.01$).

Conclusions: Research hypothesis was partially confirmed, suggesting that medical students with higher grit scores were likely to have higher empathic orientation in patient care and greater self-esteem. Conversely, those with higher degrees of grit displayed lower levels of aggression-hostility and impulsive sensation seeking. The implications of these findings for medical education are discussed.

International Journal of Medical Education, 2020, *11*, 25–30. https://www.ijme.net/archive/11/grit-and-personality-in-medical-students/

5.32   Predicting Peer Nominations: A Social
Network Approach

Barret Michalec, J. Jon Veloski, and Frederic Hafferty

Purpose: Minimal attention has been paid to what factors may predict peer nomination or how peer nominations might exhibit a clustering effect. Focusing on the homophily principle that "birds of a feather flock together," and using a social network analysis approach, the authors investigated how certain student- and/or school-based factors might predict the likelihood of peer nomination, and the clusters, if any, that occur among those nominations.

Method: In 2013, the Jefferson Longitudinal Study of Medical Education included a special instrument to evaluate peer nominations. A total of 211 (81%) of 260 graduating medical students from the Sidney Kimmel Medical College responded to the peer nomination question. Data were analyzed using a relational contingency table and an ANOVA density model.

Results: Although peer nominations did not cluster around gender, age, or class rank, those students within an accelerated program, as well as those entering certain specialties, were more likely to nominate each other. The authors suggest that clerkships in certain specialties, as well as the accelerated program, may provide structured opportunities for students to connect and integrate, and that these opportunities may have an impact on peer nomination. The findings suggest that social network analysis is a useful approach to examine various aspects of peer nomination processes.

Conclusions: The authors discuss implications regarding harnessing social cohesion within clinical clerkships, possible development of siloed departmental identity and in-group favoritism, and future research possibilities.

Academic   Medicine,   2016,   *91*(6),   847–852.   https://doi.org/10.1097/ACM.0000000000001079

5.33   Identifying Potential Engaging Leaders Within Medical Education: The Role of Positive Influence on Peers

Barret Michalec, J. Jon Veloski, Mohammadreza Hojat, and Mark L. Tykocinski

Background: Previous research has paid little to no attention toward exploring methods of identifying existing medical student leaders.

Aim: Focusing on the role of influence and employing the tenets of the engaging leadership model, this study examines demographic and academic performance-related differences of positive influencers and if students who have been peer identified as positive influencers also demonstrate high levels of genuine concern for others.

Methods: Three separate fourth-year classes were asked to designate classmates that had significant positive influences on their professional and personal development. The top 10% of those students receiving positive influence nominations were compared with the other students on demographics, academic performance, and genuine concern for others.

Results: Besides age, no demographic differences were found between positive influencers and other students. High positive influencers were not found to have higher standardized exam scores but did receive significantly higher clinical clerkship ratings. High positive influencers were found to possess a higher degree of genuine concern for others.

Conclusion: The findings lend support to (a) utilizing the engaging model to explore leaders and leadership within medical education, (b) this particular method of identifying existing medical student leaders, and (c) return the focus of leadership research to the power of influence.

Medical Teacher, 2015, *37*(7), 677–683. https://www.tandfonline.com/doi/full/10.3109/0142159X.2014.947933

5.34   How Much Do Medical Students Know About Physician Income?

Sean Nicholson

The goal of this study was to investigate how accurately medical students can estimate contemporaneous physician income, whether they make systematic errors, the determinants of any estimation errors, and how much they learn about professional income during medical school.

Method: Twenty-five cohorts of students at a large, urban, private medical school who matriculated between 1970 and 1994 were asked to estimate contemporaneous physician income in six different specialties during their first and fourth years of school.

Results: The students' income estimation errors varied systematically over time and cross section by specialty and type of student. On average, the students underestimated physician income by 15%, and the median absolute value of the estimation errors was 26% of actual income. Students were 35% more accurate when estimating market income in their fourth year relative to their first year.

Conclusion: Although this group of students were systematically uninformed about physician incomes early in their education, they learned a considerable amount during 4 years of medical school. Income estimation errors varied systematically over the time period of the study, and by the students' age, gender, specialty, and specialty plans at graduation.

The Journal of Human Resources, 2005, *40*(1), 100–114.
This abstract was written by the book editors.

5.35   Correlates of Physicians' Endorsement of the Legalization of Physician-Assisted Suicide

Karen Novielli, Mohammadreza Hojat, Thomas J. Nasca, James B. Erdmann, and J. Jon Veloski

Problem Statement and Background: Empirical studies on end-of-life care and the factors associated with legalization of physician-assisted suicide (PAS) are scarce. Our purpose was to examine the extent and correlates of physicians' endorsement of legalization of PAS.

Method: A survey was mailed in 1998 to 1272 physicians (Jefferson Medical College graduates from 1987 to 1992). Eight hundred and thirty-five responded (66%), and 830 were useable for this study.

Results: Of the respondents, 284 (34%) endorsed, 340 (41%) did not endorse, and 206 (25%) expressed no opinion about legalization of PAS. Hospital-based physicians were more likely to endorse legalization of PAS than primary care physicians. Endorsement of legalization of PAS was correlated with views about other issues in medicine and the healthcare system.

Conclusions: More empirical research is needed to understand the political, moral, and ethical contexts that frame physicians' views on PAS and to examine the impact of medical education on attitudes toward PAS.

Academic Medicine, 2000, *75*(October Supplement), S53–S55. https://doi.org/10.1097/00001888-200010001-00017

5.36   Peer Nominations as Related to Academic Attainment, Empathy, Personality, and Specialty Interest

Charles A. Pohl, Mohammadreza Hojat, and Louise Arnold

Purpose: To test the hypotheses that peer nomination is associated with measures of (1) academic performance, (2) empathy, (3) personality, and (4) specialty interest.

Method: In 2007–2008, 255 third-year medical students at Jefferson Medical College were asked to nominate classmates they considered the best in six areas of clinical and humanistic excellence. The authors compared students who received nominations with those who did not, analyzing differences in academic performance, personality factors (empathy as measured by the Jefferson Scale of Empathy and personality qualities as measured by the Zuckerman-Kuhlman Personality Questionnaire), and specialty interests.

Results: A comparison of the 155 students who received at least one peer nomination with the 100 students who received none found no significant difference in scores on objective examinations; nominated students, however, were rated significantly higher in clinical competence by faculty in six core third-year clerkships. Nominated students were also significantly more empathic and "active." In addition, a larger proportion of nominated students chose "people-oriented" (rather than "technology- or procedure-oriented") specialties.

Conclusions: These results confirmed the hypotheses that peer nomination can predict clinical competence, empathy and other positive personal qualities, and interest in people-oriented specialties. Thus, in the assessment of medical students, peer nomination holds promise as a valid indicator of positive dimensions of professionalism.

Academic Medicine, 2011, *86*(6), 747–751. https://doi.org/10.1097/ACM.0b013e318217e464

5.37   Intra- and Intercultural Comparisons of Personality Profiles of Medical Students in Argentina and the USA

Horacio J. A. Rimoldi, Roberto Raimondo, James B. Erdmann,
and Mohammadreza Hojat

This cross-cultural study was designed to examine intra- and intercultural similarities and differences on personality profiles of male and female medical students in Argentina and the USA, and to investigate psychometric properties of personality measures used in this study in medical students in Argentina. Research participants included 421 students (254 women, 167 men) from the University of El Salvador medical school, in Buenos Aires, Argentina, and 623 American medical students (207 women, 416 men) at Jefferson Medical College of Thomas Jefferson University, in the USA. Participants completed a set of personality tests measuring test-taking anxiety, loneliness experiences, external locus of control, extroversion, and neuroticism. Psychometric evidence in support of these instruments in American medical students was available. We investigated aspects of psychometrics of the translated instruments that were administered to medical students in Argentina. Results of psychometric analyses supported the validity and reliability of the translated versions of the personality tests. Statistical analyses of intracultural comparisons of medical students in Argentina showed similarities between male and female medical students in Argentina on all personality variables with the exception of test anxiety in which women scored significantly higher than men. Personality profiles of male and female medical students in the USA were also very similar with the exceptions of general anxiety test in which women scored significantly higher than men, and in the appraisal of stressful life events in which women appraised the stressful events more negatively than men. Intercultural comparisons between medical students in Argentina and the USA regardless of gender showed that students in Argentina obtained higher average scores in general anxiety, test anxiety, neuroticism, external locus of control, and perception of stressful life events. No significant difference was found between the two nationality groups on the measure of self-esteem. The results generally suggest that while statistically significant differences in personality profile exist between samples of medical students in Argentina and the USA, the underlying constructs of personality measures are similar; thus, construct validity of personality measures is relatively stable in medical students of the two countries. Given the trend toward greater globalization of medical education, it is important and timely to further study the associations between personality and academic and professional performances in medical school and beyond.

Adolescence, 2002, *37*, 477–494.
This abstract was written by the book editors.

5.38   Persistent Impostor Phenomenon is Associated with Distress in Medical Students

Susan Rosenthal, Yvette Schlussel, Mary Bit Yaden, Jennifer DeSantis, Kathryn Trayes, Charles A. Pohl, and Mohammadreza Hojat

Background and Objectives: Medical student distress and mental health needs are critical issues in undergraduate medical education. The imposter phenomenon (IP), defined as inappropriate feelings of inadequacy among high achievers, is linked to psychological distress. We investigated the prevalence of IP among first-year medical school students and its association with personality measures that affect interpersonal relationships and well-being.

Methods: Two hundred and fifty-seven students at a large urban, northeastern medical school completed the Clance Impostor Phenomenon Scale, Jefferson Scale of Empathy, Self-Compassion Scale, and Zuckerman-Kuhlman Personality Questionnaire immediately before beginning their first year of medical school. At the end of their first year, 182 of these students again completed the Clance Imposter Phenomenon Scale.

Results: Eighty-seven percent of the entering students reported high or very high degrees of IP. Students with higher IP scores had significantly lower mean scores on self-compassion, sociability, self-esteem ($p < 0.0001$ for all), and getting along with peers ($p = 0.03$). Lower IP scores were related to lower mean scores on neuroticism-anxiety and loneliness ($p < 0.001$ for both). Women obtained a higher mean IP score than men. IP scores at the end of the school year increased significantly compared with the beginning of the year ($p < 0.001$), both in frequency and intensity of IP.

Conclusion: IP was common in matriculating first-year medical students and significantly increased at year's end. Higher IP scores were significantly associated with lower scores for self-compassion, sociability, self-esteem, and higher scores on neuroticism-anxiety.

Family Medicine, 2021, 53(2), 118–122.

5.39   Income Expectations of First-Year Students at Jefferson Medical College as a Predictor of Family Practice Specialty Choice

Michael P. Rosenthal, Thane N. Turner, James J. Diamond,
and Howard K. Rabinowitz

The recent decline in the number of medical students choosing careers in the primary care specialties has engendered increasing concern that economic factors are becoming more important in influencing the career choices of medical students. In order to assess the relationship of first-year medical students' income expectations to whether they chose to specialize in family practice, the authors analyzed data from 532 graduates of Jefferson Medical College (classes of 1987–1989), using the Jefferson Longitudinal Study. At entrance to medical school, each student listed his or her initial specialty preference and future expected peak income; the determination of actual specialty choice was based on the first year of postgraduate training. Both expected peak incomes and freshman specialty choices were independent predictors of actual specialty choices. The students who entered family practice residencies had lower initial expected peak incomes than the students entering other specialties, especially the surgery specialties. In addition, according to logistic regression analysis, the students with relatively lower income expectations and a freshman preference for family practice were predicted to be nine times more likely to enter family practice residencies than students with higher income expectations and no initial family practice preference (56% versus 6%). This study suggests that a freshman's income expectation is an important predictor of family practice specialty choice, independent of age, sex, degree of indebtedness, and initial specialty preference. The authors discuss their results in light of the decline in the number of medical students choosing family practice and other primary care specialties.

Academic Medicine, 1992, *67*, 328–331.   https://doi.org/10.1097/00001888-199205000-00012

5.40   Mindfulness-Based Stress Reduction Lowers Psychological Distress in Medical Students

Steven Rosenzweig, Diane K. Reibel, Jeffrey M. Greeson, George C. Brainard, and Mohammadreza Hojat

Background: Medical students confront significant academic, psychosocial, and existential stressors throughout their training. Mindfulness-based stress reduction (MBSR) is an educational intervention designed to improve coping skills and reduce emotional distress.

Purpose: The purpose of this study was to examine the effectiveness of the MBSR intervention in a prospective, nonrandomized, cohort-controlled study.

Methods: Second-year students ($n = 140$) elected to participate in a 10-week MBSR seminar. Controls ($n = 162$) participated in a didactic seminar on complementary medicine. Profile of Mood States (POMS) was administered preintervention and postintervention.

Results: Baseline total mood disturbance (TMD) was greater in the MBSR group compared with controls (38.7 ± 33.3 vs. 28.0 ± 31.2; $p < 0.01$). Despite this initial difference, the MBSR group scored significantly lower in TMD at the completion of the intervention period (31.8 ± 33.8 vs. 38.6 ± 32.8; $p < 0.05$). Significant effects were also observed on tension-anxiety, confusion-bewilderment, fatigue-inertia, and vigor-activity subscales.

Conclusion: MBSR may be an effective stress management intervention for medical students.

Teaching and Learning in Medicine, 2003, *15*(2), 88–92. https://www.tandfonline.com/doi/abs/10.1207/S15328015TLM1502_03

5.41   The Income Expectations of Medical Students in the Time Period 1970–1980

J. Jon Veloski, Carter Zeleznik, and Mohammadreza Hojat

This study reports students' expectations of income over the past decade and analyzes the effects of factors related to these income expectations. Data collected by means of questionnaires administered to seniors at one medical school approximately 3 months prior to commencement were analyzed. The questionnaires included items dealing with the students' plans for specialty training, the number of hours per week expected to work, and the type of career planned after completion of training. The results show that graduating medical students are knowledgeable about income differentials among specialties. Women reported lower peak income expectations in each of the specialties considered, and the graduates who plan clinical careers expect higher incomes than those planning academic careers. Presently there is concern that reduced government support for education will result in student debt level changes or changes in the demographic characteristics of medical students. A long-range implication of these findings is that they provide essential baseline data needed to monitor the effects of major changes on the financing of medical education.

Proceedings of the Twentieth Annual Conference on Research in Medical Education, Washington, DC. November 1981, 61–66.

This abstract was written by the book editors.

5.42   Students' Certainty During Course Test-Taking and Performance on Clerkships and Board Exams

Carter Zeleznik, Mohammadreza Hojat, Carla E. Goepp, Peter Amadio,
Dhodanand Kowlessar, and Bette D. Borenstein

Psychometric aspects of multiple-choice tests were investigated using a confidence-weighted scoring technique. The contributions of two indices, overconfidence and under-confidence, in the prediction of subsequent academic performance of examinees were studied. A total of 444 sophomore students (entering classes of 1982 and 1983) in one medical school were asked to indicate their confidence, on a 5-point scale (100, 75, 50, 25, and 0), in the correctness of their responses to each multiple-choice item on an Introduction to Clinical Medicine examination. Examinations were scored in two ways: in the conventional way, using the total number of correct responses, and by a confidence-weighted technique based on the level of certainty indicated for each response by the examinee. Only the conventional score determined the grade; the confidence-weighted score was calculated for the purely experimental purposes of this study. Overconfidence and under-confidence indices were also calculated by using the indicated levels of certainty. Improvements in the psychometrics of the examinations were observed when confidence-weighted scores and indices of over- and under-confidence contributed significantly to predicting scores of the students on Parts I and II of the National Board of Medical Examiners examination, whereas the conventional score did not contribute to the prediction of Part II scores. Significant differences on junior clerkship examinations and ratings were observed between those who were highly overconfident and those who were slightly overconfident. The highly overconfident students also estimated higher future incomes than those who were slightly overconfident.

Journal   of   Medical   Education,   1988,   *63*,   881–891.   https://doi.
org/10.1097/00001888-198812000-00001

Chapter 6
Professionalism

Empathy, Interprofessional Collaboration, Lifelong Learning

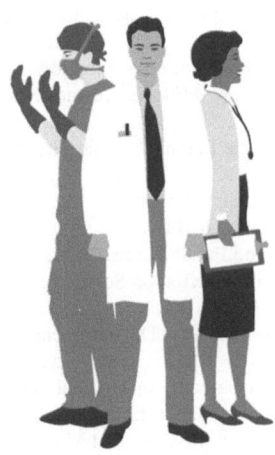

Contents

6.1   Medical Students' Self-Reported Empathy and Simulated Patients' Assessments
      of Student Empathy: An Analysis by Gender and Ethnicity.............................. 182
6.2   Comparisons of Nurses and Physicians on an Operational Measure of Empathy........ 183
6.3   Change in Empathy in Medical School... 184
6.4   Enhancing and Sustaining Empathy in Medical Students................................. 185
6.5   Patient Perceptions of Clinician's Empathy: Measurement and Psychometrics......... 186
6.6   Empathy of Medical Students and Compassionate Care for Dying Patients:
      An Assessment of "No One Dies Alone" Program.. 187
6.7   Empathy: An NP/MD Comparison.. 188
6.8   Attitudes Toward Physician-Nurse Alliance: Comparisons of Medical and Nursing
      Students.. 189
6.9   Psychometric Properties of an Attitude Scale Measuring Physician-Nurse
      Collaboration.. 190
6.10 An Instrument for Measuring Pharmacist and Physician Attitudes Toward
      Collaboration: Preliminary Psychometric Data.. 191
6.11 Eleven Years of Data on the Jefferson Scale of Empathy-Medical Student Version
      (JSE-S): Proxy Norm Data and Tentative Cutoff Scores................................. 192
6.12 Letter to the Editor: In Reply to Quinn and Zelenski................................. 193
6.13 What Matters More About the Interpersonal Reactivity Index and the Jefferson
      Scale of Empathy? Their Underlying Constructs or Their Relationships
      with Pertinent Measures of Clinical Competence and Patient Outcomes................ 194

6.14   Physician Empathy in Medical Education and Practice: Experience
        with the Jefferson Scale of Physician Empathy.. 195
6.15   Empathy in Medical Students as Related to Academic Performance, Clinical
        Competence, and Gender.. 196
6.16   Comparisons of American, Israeli, Italian, and Mexican Physicians and Nurses
        on the Total and Factor Scores of the Jefferson Scale of Attitudes Toward
        Physician-Nurse Collaborative Relationships.. 197
6.17   The Jefferson Scale of Physician Empathy: Further Psychometric Data
        and Differences by Gender and Specialty at Item Level................................... 198
6.18   Physician Empathy: Definition, Components, Measurement, and Relationship
        to Gender and Specialty... 199
6.19   Rebuttals to Critics of Studies of the Decline of Empathy.............................. 200
6.20   Developing an Instrument to Measure Attitudes Toward Nurses: Preliminary
        Psychometric Findings... 201
6.21   Exploration and Confirmation of the Latent Variable Structure of the Jefferson
        Scale of Empathy... 202
6.22   The Jefferson Scale of Empathy (JSE): An Update... 203
6.23   Editorial: Empathy and Health Care Quality.. 204
6.24   Empathy in Medical Education and Patient Care.. 205
6.25   Relationships Between Scores of the Jefferson Scale of Physician Empathy (JSPE)
        and the Interpersonal Reactivity Index (IRI)... 206
6.26   The Jefferson Scale of Physician Empathy: Development and Preliminary
        Psychometric Data.. 207
6.27   An Empirical Study of Decline in Empathy in Medical School.......................... 208
6.28   Attitudes Toward Physician-Nurse Collaboration: A Cross-cultural Study of Male
        and Female Physicians and Nurses in the USA and Mexico.............................. 209
6.29   An Operational Measure of Physician Lifelong Learning: Its Development,
        Components, and Preliminary Psychometric Data... 210
6.30   Psychometrics of the Scale of Attitudes Toward Physician-Pharmacist
        Collaboration: A Study with Medical Students... 211
6.31   Measurement and Correlates of Physicians' Lifelong Learning......................... 212
6.32   Physician Lifelong Learning: Conceptualization, Measurement, and Correlates
        in Full-Time Clinicians and Academic Clinicians... 213
6.33   Assessing Physicians' Orientation Toward Lifelong Learning........................... 214
6.34   The Jefferson Scale of Attitudes Toward Interprofessional Collaboration
        (JEFFSATIC): Development and Multi-institution Psychometric Data............... 215
6.35   Empathy in Medical Students as Related to Specialty Interest, Personality,
        and Perceptions of Mother and Father... 216
6.36   Enhancing Student Empathetic Engagement, History-Taking, and Communication
        Skills During Electronic Medical Record Use in Patient Care.......................... 217
6.37   Assessment of Empathy in Different Years of Internal Medicine Training........... 218
6.38   Evaluating the Relationship Between Participation in Student-Run Free Clinics
        and Changes in Empathy in Medical Students... 219
6.39   Measuring Professionalism: A Review of Studies with Instruments Reported
        in the Literature Between 1982 and 2002... 220
6.40   Linguistic Analysis of Empathy in Medical School Admission Essays................ 221

Abstract

- The data in the Jefferson Longitudinal Study served as the foundation for the development and psychometric analyses of core measures of professionalism in medicine, such as clinical empathy in patient care, interprofessional collaboration, and lifelong learning. This section includes highlights of findings on these measures.
- The Jefferson Scale of Empathy, used worldwide, has been translated into 67 languages, and used in more than 85 countries. The other instruments on interprofessional collaboration and lifelong learning have also been translated into other languages.
- Studies with medical and other health professions students suggest significant correlations between these measures of professionalism.
- Medical students who volunteered to participate in a program to provide compassionate care companionship to terminally ill and lonely patients scored higher than non-volunteers on clinical empathy. Also, comparing volunteer and non-volunteer students to serve homeless and indigent patients in a student-run free clinic showed that orientation toward empathy in patient care declined in the non-volunteer group; however, no such empathy decline was observed in the volunteer group.
- Medical students' empathic orientation could be predicted from medical school admission essays based on the language used in application essays.
- A simple intervention on proper use of electronic medical records in patient care could help to improve medical students' empathy, history-taking skills, and communication skills.
- Higher scores on clinical empathy were associated with students' interest in people-oriented (as opposed to technology-oriented) specialties, higher level of satisfaction with early maternal relationships, higher scores on sociability, and lower scores on aggression-hostility.
- Comparisons of physicians and nurses in the USA, Mexico, Israel, and Italy on their attitudes toward physician-nurse collaboration showed inter- and intracultural similarities and differences consistent with the social role theory and the principle of least interest (e.g., greater power position, less inclination for collaborative relationship).

Keywords Cross-cultural comparisons · Dying patient · Empathy and academic performance · Empathy and patient outcomes · Empathy and specialty interest · Erosion of empathy · Enhancement of empathy · Interprofessional collaboration and teamwork · Jefferson Scale of Empathy (JSE) · Lifelong learning · Measures of professionalism · Objective Structured Clinical Examination (OSCE) · Patient perceptions · Physician-nurse collaboration · Physician-pharmacist collaboration · Simulated patient · Standardized patient · Student-run free clinic · Sustaining empathy · Volunteerism

6.1   Medical Students' Self-Reported Empathy and Simulated Patients' Assessments of Student Empathy: An Analysis by Gender and Ethnicity

Katherine Berg, Joseph F. Majdan, Dale Berg, J. Jon Veloski,
and Mohammadreza Hojat

Purpose: To examine the contribution of students' gender and ethnicity to assessments by simulated patients (SPs) of medical students' empathy, and to compare the results with students' self-assessments of their own empathy.

Method: In 2008, the authors used three different tools to assess the empathy of 248 third-year medical students. Students completed the Jefferson Scale of Physician Empathy (JSPE), and SPs completed the Jefferson Scale of Patient Perceptions of Physician Empathy (JSPPPE) and a global rating of empathy (GRE) in 10 Objective Structured Clinical Examination (OSCE) encounters.

Results: Of the 248 students who completed an end-of-third-year OSCE, 176 (71%) also completed the JSPE. Results showed that women scored higher than men on all three measures of empathy. The authors detected no significant difference between white and Asian-American students on their self-report JSPE scores. However, the SPs' assessments on the JSPPPE and on the GRE were significantly lower, indicating less empathy, for Asian-American students.

Conclusions: A tool for SPs to assess students' empathy during an OSCE could be helpful for unmasking some deficits in empathy in students during the third year of medical school. Because the authors found no significant differences on self-reported empathy, the differences they observed in the SPs' assessments of white and Asian-American students were unexpected and need further exploration. These findings call for investigation into the reasons for such differences so that OSCEs and other examinations comply with the guidelines for fairness in educational and psychological testing as recommended by professional testing organizations.

Academic   Medicine,   2011,   *86*,   984–988.   https://doi.org/10.1097/
ACM.0b013e3182224f1f

6.2   Comparisons of Nurses and Physicians on an Operational Measure of Empathy

Sylvia K. Fields, Mohammadreza Hojat, Joseph S. Gonnella,
Salvatore Mangione, Gregory C. Kane, and Mike Magee

In view of many changes taking place in today's healthcare marketplace, the theme of empathy in health provider-patient relations needs to be revisited. It has been proposed that patients benefit when all members of the healthcare team provide empathic care. Despite the role of empathy in patient outcomes, empirical research on empathy among health professionals is scarce partly because of a lack of a psychometrically sound tool to measure it. In this study, we briefly describe the development and validation of the Jefferson Scale of Physician Empathy (JSPE), an instrument that was specifically developed to measure empathy among health professionals (20 Likert-type items). The purpose of this study was to compare nurses and physicians on their responses to the JSPE. Study participants were 56 female registered nurses and 42 female physicians in the internal medicine postgraduate medical education program at Thomas Jefferson University Hospital. The reliability coefficients (Cronbach's coefficient alpha) were 0.87 for the nurses and 0.89 for physicians. Results of t-test showed no significant difference between nurses and physicians on total scores of the JSPE; however, multivariate analyses of variance indicated statistically significant differences between the two groups on 5 of 20 items of the JSPE. Findings suggest that the JSPE is a reliable research tool that can be used to assess empathy among health professionals including nurses.

Evaluation & The Health Professions, 2004, 27(1), 80–94.

6.3   Change in Empathy in Medical School

Mohammadreza Hojat

Controversial findings from a published study in *Medical Education* suggest that as students progressed through medical school their empathy declined when measured by the Jefferson Scale of Empathy (JSE), but improved when measured by another instrument developed for administration to the general population (Questionnaire of Cognitive and Affective Empathy). The authors of that study challenged the findings on erosion of empathy in medical students reported for the first time by us and reported subsequently in another study by our team as well as others. We argued that the sensitivity, specificity, and utility of empathy-measuring instruments can explain the inconsistent results.

First, differences in a germane definition of empathy in the context of patient care determine the content validity of the test. In conceptualization of empathy in patient care, we made a distinction between cognition and affect, and between understanding and feeling. With regard to consequential outcomes of cognition vs. affect, and of understanding vs. feeling in clinical encounters, we deliberately defined empathy as predominantly a cognitive (rather than an affective) attribute to understand (rather than to feel) patients' pain and suffering. Thus, the JSE could be more sensitive in detecting changes in clinical empathy because it was developed based on a pertinent cognitive conceptualization of empathy.

Second, the target population for the instrument determines the specificity of the language used in the test (face validity). The JSE is more content specific and context relevant to patient care because it was developed for administration to health professions students and practitioners. In addition, its psychometrics have been supported exclusively in the target population of health professions students and practitioners. This is not the case with other empathy-measuring instruments which were developed for administration to the general population.

Third, the utilization of an empathy-measuring instrument in health professions education and patient care is determined by its significant link to pertinent criterion measures of clinical competence and tangible patient outcomes. Such validity evidence is readily available for the JSE in predicting clinical competence in medical students and positive patient outcomes in diabetic patients.

Thus, differences in sensitivity, specificity, and utility of the JSE compared to other empathy-measuring instruments that were developed for administration to the general population can provide plausible explanation for inconsistent findings on decline in empathy in medical students.

Medical Education (Letter to the Editor), 2018, *52*, 456–457. https://doi.org/10.1111/medu.13497
This abstract was written by the book editors.

6.4   Enhancing and Sustaining Empathy in Medical Students

Mohammadreza Hojat, David Axelrod, John Spandorfer,
and Salvatore Mangione

Background: Empathy is an important component of physician competence that needs to be enhanced.

Aim: To test the hypotheses that medical students' empathy can be enhanced and sustained by targeted activities.

Methods: This was a two-phase study in which 248 medical students participated. In Phase 1, students in the experimental group watched and discussed video clips of patient encounters meant to enhance empathic understanding; those in the control group watched a documentary film. Ten weeks later in Phase 2 of the study, students who were in the experimental group were divided into two groups. One group attended a lecture on empathy in patient care, and the other plus the control group watched a movie about racism. The Jefferson Scale of Empathy (JSE) was administered pre-post in Phase 1 and posttest in Phase 2.

Results: In Phase 1, the JSE mean score for the experimental group improved significantly ($p < 0.01$); no change in the JSE scores was observed in the control group. In Phase 2, the JSE mean score improvement was sustained in the group that attended the lecture, but not in the other group. No change in empathy was noticed in the control group.

Conclusion: Research hypotheses were confirmed.

Medical Teacher, 2013, *35*(12), 996–1001. https://www.tandfonline.com/doi/full/1 0.3109/0142159X.2013.802300

6.5   Patient Perceptions of Clinician's Empathy: Measurement and Psychometrics

Mohammadreza Hojat, Jennifer DeSantis, and Joseph S. Gonnella

The prominence of reciprocal understanding in patient-doctor empathic engagement implies that patient perception of clinician's empathy has an important role in the assessment of the patient-clinician relationship. In response to a need for an assessment tool to measure patient's views of clinician empathy, we developed a brief (5-item) instrument, *the Jefferson Scale of Patient Perceptions of Physician Empathy (JSPPPE)*. This review article reports evidence in support of the validity and reliability of the JSPPPE.

Journal of Patient Experience, 2017, 4(2), 78–83.

6.6   Empathy of Medical Students and Compassionate Care for Dying Patients: An Assessment of "No One Dies Alone" Program

Mohammadreza Hojat, Jennifer DeSantis, David B. Ney,
and Hannah DeCleene-Do

The "No One Dies Alone" (NODA) program was initiated to provide compassionate companions to the bedside of dying patients. This study was designed to test the following hypotheses: (1) Empathy scores would be higher among medical students who volunteered to participate in the NODA program than non-volunteers. (2) Spending time with dying patients would enhance empathy in medical students. Study sample included 525 first- and second-year medical students, 54 of whom volunteered to participate in the NODA program. Of these volunteers, 26 had the opportunity to visit a dying patient (experimental group), and 28 did not, due to scheduling conflicts (volunteer control group). The rest of the sample ($n = 471$) comprised the "non-volunteer control group." Comparisons of the aforementioned groups on scores of the Jefferson Scale of Empathy confirmed the first research hypothesis ($p < 0.05$, Cohen's $d = 0.37$); the second hypothesis was not confirmed. This study has implications for the assessment of empathy in physicians in training, and timely for recruiting compassionate companion volunteers (armed with personal protective equipment) at the bedside of lonely dying patients infected by COVID-19.

Journal of Patient Experience, 2020, *7*(6), 1164–1168.

6.7   Empathy: An NP/MD Comparison

Mohammadreza Hojat, Sylvia K. Fields, and Joseph S. Gonnella

The Jefferson Scale of Physician Empathy (JSPE, 20 Likert-type items) was administered to 32 female nurse practitioners, 37 female pediatricians, and 33 female physicians in hospital-based specialties (anesthesiology, pathology, radiology). Nurse practitioners and pediatricians obtained higher JSPE mean scores than physicians in hospital-based specialties.

The Nurse Practitioner, 2003, *28*(4), 45–47. https://journals.lww.com/tnpj/fulltext/2003/04000/empathy__an_np_md_comparison.10.aspx

6.8   Attitudes Toward Physician-Nurse Alliance: Comparisons of Medical and Nursing Students

Mohammadreza Hojat, Sylvia K. Fields, Susan L. Rattner, Margaret Griffiths, Mitchell J. M. Cohen, and James D. Plumb

This study was undertaken to examine empirically the similarities and differences between medical and nursing students in their attitudes toward physician-nurse alliances upon entry into their respective professional curricula.

The participants were 408 medical students (208 first year, 200 second year) and 149 nursing students (64 first year, 85 second year) representing 90% and 89%, respectively, of students in their corresponding classes.

The findings suggest considerable attitudinal congruities among medical and nursing students as they begin their professional education. Overall the medical students hold to the traditional views of physician authority and medical responsibility in these areas to a higher degree than the nursing students, although the data suggest more concordance and recognition of professionalism in nursing than would have been seen in the past. The findings of this study provide useful information regarding the areas of focus for interdisciplinary educational programs.

Academic Medicine, 1997, *72*(Supplement), S1–S3. https://doi.org/10.1097/00001888-199710001-00001

6.9   Psychometric Properties of an Attitude Scale Measuring Physician-Nurse Collaboration

Mohammadreza Hojat, Sylvia K. Fields, J. Jon Veloski, Margaret Griffiths, Mitchell J. M. Cohen, and James D. Plumb

This study examined the psychometric properties of an assessment tool for measuring attitudes toward physician-nurse collaboration. A survey addressing the areas of responsibility, expectations, shared learning, decision-making, authority, and autonomy was administered to first-year medical and nursing students. Factor analysis of the survey indicated that the survey measured four underlying constructs of shared education and collaborative relationships, caring as opposed to curing, nurse's autonomy, and physician's authority. A scale was developed in which 15 items of the survey with large factor loadings were included. The alpha reliability estimates of the scale for medical and nursing students were 0.84 and 0.85, respectively. The mean of the scale was significantly higher for nursing than medical students. Results supported the construct validity and reliability of the scale. This scale can be used to evaluate the effectiveness of programs developed to foster physician-nurse collaboration and to study group differences on attitudes toward interpersonal collaboration.

Evaluation & The Health Professions, 1999, 22(2), 208–220.

Copyright©   1999.   Sage   Publishing.   https://journals.sagepub.com/ doi/10.1177/01632789922034275

6.10   An Instrument for Measuring Pharmacist and Physician Attitudes Toward Collaboration: Preliminary Psychometric Data

Mohammadreza Hojat and Joseph S. Gonnella

This study was designed to develop an instrument for measuring attitudes toward pharmacist-physician collaborative relationships for administration to practicing pharmacists and physicians, as well as to students in pharmacy and medical schools. Based on a review of literature, a preliminary version of an instrument was developed (30 items), and through a pilot study of face validity and content validity with 12 pharmacists and 10 physicians, 18 items were chosen for quantitative analyses. We asked 88 respondents (61 pharmacists, 27 physicians) to judge the relevance, clarity, and representativeness of each item to the concept of pharmacist-physician collaborative relationships. Sixteen items with a relevancy endorsement greater than 85% and significant item-total score correlations were retained. The following underlying constructs emerged from factor analysis: "collaboration and teamwork," "accountability," "overlapping responsibility," and "authority." These factors supported the multidimensionality and construct validity of the instrument. No gender difference was observed; however, pharmacists scored higher than physicians on the total score of the instrument. The Cronbach's coefficient alpha was 0.81 for pharmacists, 0.92 for physicians, and 0.87 for the combined sample. Encouraged by these preliminary findings, we plan to undertake further research to examine the instrument's psychometric properties including criterion-related and predictive validities with larger and more representative samples of pharmacists, physicians, and students in pharmacy and medical schools.

Journal of Interprofessional Care, 2011, 25(1), 66–72. https://www.tandfonline.com/doi/full/10.3109/13561820.2010.483368

6.11 Eleven Years of Data on the Jefferson Scale of Empathy-Medical Student Version (JSE-S): Proxy Norm Data and Tentative Cutoff Scores

Mohammadreza Hojat and Joseph S. Gonnella

Objective: This study was designed to provide typical descriptive statistics, score distributions, and percentile ranks of the Jefferson Scale of Empathy-Medical Student version (JSE-S) of male and female medical school matriculants to serve as proxy norm data and tentative cutoff scores.

Subjects and Methods: The participants were 2637 students (1336 women and 1301 men) who matriculated at Sidney Kimmel (formerly Jefferson) Medical College between 2002 and 2012, and completed the JSE at the beginning of medical school. Information extracted from descriptive statistics, score distributions, and percentile ranks for male and female matriculants was used to develop proxy norm data and tentative cutoff scores.

Results: The score distributions of the JSE tended to be moderately skewed and platykurtic. Women obtained a significantly higher mean score (116.2 ± 9.7) than men (112.3 ± 10.8) on the JSE-S ($t2,635 = 9.9$, $p < 0.01$). It was suggested that percentile ranks can be used as proxy norm data. The tentative cutoff score to identify low scorers was ≤ 95 for men and ≤ 100 for women.

Conclusions: Our findings provide norm data and cutoff scores for admission decisions under certain conditions and for identifying students in need of enhancing their empathy.

Medical Principles and Practice: International Journal of the Kuwait University, Health Science Centre, 2015, 24, 344–350.

6.12   Letter to the Editor: In Reply to Quinn and Zelenski

Mohammadreza Hojat and Joseph S. Gonnella

In response to a misinterpretation of our views expressed in an invited commentary on empathy in medical education and patient care, we indicated that the following points were overlooked: In the context of patient care, we made a distinction between empathy (defined as a cognitive attribute involving understanding) and sympathy (defined as an emotional reaction involving intense feelings). The afore-mentioned distinctions imply different consequences in patient care, where abundance of empathy, due to its cognitive nature and mental mechanism of understanding, would likely to be always beneficial. In contrast, sympathy in excess, due to its emotional nature and mental mechanism of intense feeling, can be overwhelming, and thus likely to be detrimental to both the clinician (e.g., leading to exhaustion and burnout) and the patient (e.g., leading to emotional dependency, and obstacle to objective clinical decisions). We therefore concluded that in a clinical context, empathy binds patients and clinicians together, whereas sympathy in excess blinds them to objectivity which is an essential component of patient care. We suggested that both empathic understanding and affective sympathy are relevant to patient care, but for optimal patient outcomes, empathy (understanding) must be maximized, but sympathy (intense emotions) must be regulated.

Academic Medicine (Letter to the Editor), 2017, *92*(9), 1219.
   This abstract was written by the book editors.

6.13   What Matters More About the Interpersonal Reactivity Index and the Jefferson Scale of Empathy? Their Underlying Constructs or Their Relationships with Pertinent Measures of Clinical Competence and Patient Outcomes

Mohammadreza Hojat and Joseph S. Gonnella

In their study published in this issue of Academic Medicine, Costa and colleagues confirmed the underlying constructs of the Interpersonal Reactivity Index (IRI) and the Jefferson Scale of Empathy (JSE) in medical students. The authors of this Commentary propose that in comparing two instruments that both purport to measure empathy, researchers or test users must pay close attention to the target populations, the conceptualizations of empathy, and the validity evidence in relation to pertinent criterion measures. The Commentary's authors draw attention to the fact that the IRI was developed for administration to the general population, whereas the JSE was developed specifically for administration to students and practitioners of health professions. Also, the author of the IRI conceptualized empathy as a combination of cognitive and emotional attributes, whereas the authors of the JSE defined empathy as a predominantly cognitive attribute. These differences are reflected in the content of the items, which determines the underlying constructs of the two instruments. The Commentary authors suggest that any empathy-measuring instrument in the context of health professions education and patient care requires the crucial evidence of significant relationships with indicators of clinical competence and positive patient outcomes. Such validity evidence is readily available for the JSE, and the Commentary authors recommend that researchers make efforts to provide pertinent validity support for any other instrument measuring empathy in health professionals in training and in practice.

Academic Medicine (Invited Commentary), 2017, *92*(6), 743–745. https://doi.org/10.1097/ACM.0000000000001424

6.14　Physician Empathy in Medical Education and Practice: Experience with the Jefferson Scale of Physician Empathy

Mohammadreza Hojat, Joseph S. Gonnella, Salvatore Mangione,
Thomas J. Nasca, and Mike Magee

Despite the importance of physician empathy in patient care, empirical investigation on the topic is scarce because of conceptual ambiguity and a lack of a psychometrically sound tool for measuring physician empathy. In this study we describe different conceptual views of empathy, draw a distinction between empathy and sympathy, and define physician empathy. We also describe the development and psychometric properties (i.e., validity and reliability) of the Jefferson Scale of Physician Empathy (JSPE), a brief research tool (20 Likert-type items) that we developed as a response to the need for an operational measure of physician empathy. We outline an agenda for future research on physician empathy. We conclude that research regarding physician empathy is crucial considering the rapid developments in biotechnology and the current trend toward market-driven, corporate medicine, which strain the physician-patient relationships.

Seminars in Integrative Medicine, 2003, *1*(1), 25–41.

6.15   Empathy in Medical Students as Related to Academic Performance, Clinical Competence, and Gender

Mohammadreza Hojat, Joseph S. Gonnella, Salvatore Mangione,
Thomas J. Nasca, J. Jon Veloski, James B. Erdmann, Clara A. Callahan,
and Mike Magee

Context: Empathy is a major component of patient-physician relationships, and the cultivation and evaluation of empathy is a learning objective for all American medical schools as proposed by the Association of American Medical Colleges (AAMC). It is important to address the measurement of empathy, its development, and its correlates in medical schools.

Objectives: We designed this study to test two hypotheses: (1) Medical students with higher empathy scores would obtain higher ratings of clinical competence in core clinical clerkships. (2) Women would obtain higher empathy scores than men.

Materials and Subjects: A 20-item empathy scale developed by the authors (Jefferson Scale of Physician Empathy) was completed by 371 third-year medical students (198 men, 173 women).

Methods: Associations between empathy scores and ratings of clinical competence in six core clerkships, gender, and performance on objective examinations were studied by using *t*-test, analysis of variance, and correlation coefficients.

Results: Both research hypotheses were confirmed. Empathy scores were associated with ratings of clinical competence and gender, but not with performance on objective examinations such as the Medical College Admission Test (MCAT), and Steps 1 and 2 of the United States Medical Licensing Examinations (USMLE).

Conclusions: Empathy scores are associated with gender and ratings of clinical competence in medical school. It is important to further examine educational and clinical correlates of empathy, as well as stability and changes in empathy at different stages of undergraduate and graduate medical education in future research.

Medical Education, 2002, *36*(6), 522–527. https://onlinelibrary.wiley.com/doi/full/10.1046/j.1365-2923.2002.01234.x

6.16   Comparisons of American, Israeli, Italian, and Mexican Physicians and Nurses on the Total and Factor Scores of the Jefferson Scale of Attitudes Toward Physician-Nurse Collaborative Relationships

Mohammadreza Hojat, Joseph S. Gonnella, Thomas J. Nasca, Sylvia K. Fields, Americo Cicchetti, Alessandra Lo Scalzo, Francesco Taroni, Anna Maria Vicenza Amicosante, Manuela Macinati, Massimo Tangucci, Carlo Liva, Gualtiero Ricciardi, Shmuel Eidelman, Hanna Admi, Hana Geva, Tanya Mashiach, Gideon Alroy, Adelina Alcorta-Gonzalez, David Ibarra, and Antonio Torres-Ruiz

This cross-cultural study was designed to compare the attitudes of physicians and nurses toward physician-nurse collaboration in the USA, Israel, Italy, and Mexico. Total participants were 2522 physicians and nurses who completed the Jefferson Scale of Attitudes Toward Physician-Nurse Collaboration (15 Likert-type items). They were compared on the total scores and four factors of the Jefferson Scale (shared education and teamwork, caring as opposed to curing, nurses' autonomy, physicians' dominance). Results showed inter- and intracultural similarities and differences among the study groups providing support for the social role theory and the principle of least interest in interprofessional relationships. Implications for promoting physician-nurse education and interprofessional collaboration are discussed.

International Journal of Nursing Studies, 2003, *40*(4), 427–435.
Reprinted with permission from Elsevier.

6.17   The Jefferson Scale of Physician Empathy: Further Psychometric Data and Differences by Gender and Specialty at Item Level

Mohammadreza Hojat, Joseph S. Gonnella, Thomas J. Nasca,
Salvatore Mangione, J. Jon Veloski, and Michael Magee

Objective: This study was designed to investigate the psychometric properties of individual items of the Jefferson Scale of Physician Empathy by examining differences between men and women and between physicians in the "people-oriented" and "technology-oriented" specialties.

Method: The Jefferson Scale of Physician Empathy (20 Likert-type items) was mailed to 1007 physicians affiliated with the Jefferson Health System in the greater Philadelphia region; 704 (70%) responded.

Results: Descriptive statistics for items and item-total score correlations were reported. Women scored higher than men on 6 items. Physicians in the "people-oriented" specialties scored significantly higher than those in "technology-oriented" specialties on 11 items.

Conclusions: Findings provided further evidence in support of the psychometric properties of the Scale. Group differences observed in this study indicate that some aspects of empathy are more related than others to physician's gender and specialty.

Academic Medicine, 2002, 77(10), S58–S60. https://doi.org/10.1097/00001888-200210001-00019

6.18　Physician Empathy: Definition, Components, Measurement, and Relationship to Gender and Specialty

Mohammadreza Hojat, Joseph S. Gonnella, Thomas J. Nasca, Salvatore Mangione, Michael J. Vergare, and Michael Magee

Objective: There is a dearth of empirical research on physician empathy despite its mediating role in patient-physician relationships and clinical outcomes. This study was designed to investigate the components of physician empathy, its measurement properties, and group differences in empathy scores.

Method: A revised version of the Jefferson Scale of Physician Empathy (with 20 Likert-type items) was mailed to 1007 physicians affiliated with the Jefferson Health System in the greater Philadelphia region; 704 (70%) responded. Construct validity, reliability of the empathy scale, and differences on mean empathy scores by physicians' gender and specialty were examined.

Results: Three meaningful factors emerged (perspective taking, compassionate care, and standing in the patient's shoes) to provide support for the construct validity of the empathy scale, which was also found to be internally consistent with relatively stable scores over time. Women scored higher than men to a degree that was nearly significant with control for gender, and psychiatrists scored a mean empathy rating that was significantly higher than that of physicians specializing in anesthesiology, orthopedic surgery, neurosurgery, radiology, cardiovascular surgery, obstetrics and gynecology, and general surgery. No significant difference was observed on empathy scores among physicians specializing in psychiatry, internal medicine, pediatrics, emergency medicine, and family medicine.

Conclusions: Empathy is a multidimensional concept that varies among physicians and can be measured with a psychometrically sound tool. Implications for specialty selection and career counseling are discussed.

American Journal of Psychiatry, 2002, *159*(9), 1563–1569.

6.19   Rebuttals to Critics of Studies of the Decline of Empathy

Mohammadreza Hojat, Joseph S. Gonnella, and J. Jon Veloski

This study is a rebuttal to critics that findings on decline in empathy in medical students have been greatly exaggerated. We refuted by indicating that first, although empathy is considered by the critics as an elusive concept, in the context of patient care we defined empathy as a predominantly *cognitive* attribute that involves an *understanding* of patients' experiences, concerns, and perspectives combined with a capacity to *communicate* this understanding and an *intention to help*.

Second, the critics who raised concern about the validity of the Jefferson Scale of Empathy (JSE) failed to recognize the extensive literature and its psychometrics. Because of the strong evidence in support of its validity and reliability, the JSE has been broadly used by researchers in the USA and abroad. In addition, a relationship between physicians' JSE scores and scores on the Jefferson Scale of Patient Perception of Physician Empathy has been reported. Furthermore, we reported a strong link between physicians' scores on the JSE and clinical outcomes of their diabetic patients.

Finally, to address the issue of clinical or practical significance of the findings, we reported the effect size of the declined empathy scores in medical students, which yields a "scale-free" and operationally defined measure of changes in empathy scores. The effect sizes for declining empathy in our studies ranged from 0.29 to 0.64.

Critical review of the literature on important issues, such as empathy in physicians in training, can potentially make valuable contributions when the criticism is well founded. We firmly stand behind our concluding remarks that erosion of empathy observed in our studies is not only statistically significant but also of practical importance that must not be ignored.

Academic Medicine, 2010, *85*(12), 1812; (Letter to the Editor), 1813–1814. https://journals.lww.com/academicmedicine/Fulltext/2010/12000/Rebuttals_to_Critics_of_Studies_of_the_Decline_of.2.aspx

6.20 Developing an Instrument to Measure Attitudes Toward Nurses: Preliminary Psychometric Findings

Mohammadreza Hojat and Mary W. Herman

Although many doctors and nurses presumably develop good working relationships, substantial problems are frequently reported. There is a large body of reports on physicians' attitudes toward perceptions of nurses, but no systematic attempt has been made to develop a psychometrically sound instrument to measure attitudes toward nurses. This study reports steps in developing such an instrument and its psychometric characteristics. Based on a review of the literature, a preliminary list of 59 statements of attitudes toward nurses was prepared and subsequently reviewed by 26 medical educators, nurses, and physicians. Twenty-five statements were judged to have adequate face validity and were included in a preliminary version of a questionnaire using a 4-point Likert-type format. Quantitative analyses were performed on the responses in two studies with medical students. In the first study, 67 freshmen and sophomore medical students participated. In this sample those who participated in a summer program, working with nurses to observe nurses' contributions to patient care, scored the highest mean score on the 20-item Attitudes Toward Nurses instrument ($M = 64$). Those who volunteered for the program and were not selected to actually participate in the program obtained the next highest mean score ($M = 61.79$), and finally, those who did not volunteer to participate in the program obtained the lowest mean score ($M = 58.28$). The difference between non-volunteer and the two other groups was statistically significant ($F(2,64) = 3.73, p < 0.05$). In another study, 15 freshman students completed the Attitudes Toward Nurses instrument before and immediately after the program, where significant improvement was observed in the posttest ($t(14) = 2.61, p < 0.05$). Scores of the 20 statements (items) yielded a significant and positive correlation with the total score. Statistical analyses of the 20-item version of the scale supported its psychometric characteristics.

Psychological Reports, 1985, *56*, 571–579.

6.21   Exploration and Confirmation of the Latent Variable Structure of the Jefferson Scale of Empathy

Mohammadreza Hojat and Marianna LaNoue

Objectives: To reaffirm the underlying components of the JSE by using exploratory factor analysis (EFA), and to confirm its latent variable structure by using confirmatory factor analysis (CFA).

Methods: Research participants included 2612 medical students who entered Jefferson Medical College between 2002 and 2012. This sample was divided into two groups: matriculants between 2002 and 2007 ($n = 1380$) and between 2008 and 2012 ($n = 1232$). Data for 2002–2007 matriculants were subjected to EFA (principal component factor extraction), and data for matriculants of 2008–2012 were used for CFA (structural equation modeling, and root mean square error for approximation).

Results: The EFA resulted in three factors: "perspective taking," "compassionate care," and "walking in patient's shoes" replicating the 3-factor model reported in most of the previous studies. The CFA showed that the 3-factor model was an acceptable fit, thus confirming the latent variable structure that emerged in the EFA. Corrected item-total score correlations for the total sample were all positive and statistically significant, ranging from 0.13 to 0.61 with a median of 0.44 ($p < 0.01$). The item discrimination effect size indices (contrasting item mean scores for the top-third versus bottom-third JSE scorers) ranged from 0.50 to 1.4 indicating that the differences in item mean scores between top and bottom scorers on the JSE were of practical importance. Cronbach's alpha coefficient of the JSE for the total sample was 0.80, ranging from 0.75 to 0.84 for matriculants of different years.

Conclusions: Findings provided further support for underlying constructs of the JSE, adding to its credibility.

International Journal of Medical Education, 2014, *5*, 73–81. https://www.ijme.net/archive/5/latent-variable-structure-of-jse/?ref=linkout

6.22   The Jefferson Scale of Empathy (JSE): An Update

Mohammadreza Hojat, Daniel Z. Louis, Kaye Maxwell, and Joseph S. Gonnella

We briefly described the three versions of the Jefferson Scale of Empathy (JSE) developed for administration to physicians and other healthcare providers, medical students, and health professions students other than medical students. Selected findings from studies in which the JSE was used on gender difference (in favor of women) and specialty interest (in favor of primary care versus hospital-based specialties) are discussed. Also, significant associations observed between scores of the JSE and higher ratings of clinical competent in medical students (given by medical school faculty in six core clerkships in the third year of medical school), popularity in medical students (measured by peer nomination method), simulated patients' assessment of medical students (by Objective Structured Clinical Examinations), patient perceptions of physician empathy, and patient outcomes (pertinent laboratory test results) were reported. In addition, findings on decline in empathy starting in third year of medical school, possibility of enhancement of empathy by targeted educational workshops/remedies, and distinctions between empathy and sympathy are briefly discussed.

Population Health Matters (Formerly Health Policy Newsletter), 2011, 24(2), 5–6.
  This abstract was written by the book editors.

6.23   Editorial: Empathy and Health Care Quality

Mohammadreza Hojat, Daniel Z. Louis, Vittorio Maio, and Joseph S. Gonnella

Empathy defined as a predominantly cognitive (as opposed to an affective) attribute makes a distinction between empathy (a cognitive attribute) and sympathy (an affective response). Such a distinction is important in the context of patient care because an overabundance of sympathy, due to its affective nature, can be detrimental to patients as well as physicians (interferes with objectivity in clinical decisions, leads to exhaustion and burnout). However, empathy due to its cognitive nature, even in excess, is always beneficial to patient care. This definition implies that an empathic engagement revolves around reciprocity and mutual understanding. Such a reciprocal relationship evokes "psycho-socio-bio-neurological" responses, providing plausible explanations for the observed relationship between physician empathy and patient outcomes. At the psychosocial level, empathic engagement lays the foundation for a trusting relationship. Constraints in communication will diminish when a trusting relationship is formed; consequently a trusting relationship will be developed that leads to a more accurate diagnosis and greater compliance, ultimately resulting in a better quality care. At the bio-neurological level, empathic engagement is analogous to a synchronized dance between involved parties, which is orchestrated by bio-neurological markers. In addition, a set of neurons, known as the mirror neuron system (MNS), is discharged when observing another person performing a goal-directed act, as if the observer is performing the act. This leads to more empathic engagement. We conclude that empathy must be considered as an important component of physician competence. Therefore, leaders in the healthcare institutions and academic medical centers must act upon a mandate to take one step further than just declaring the desirability of empathic engagement in patient care. They must implement and rigorously assess targeted educational programs to enhance empathy in physicians in training and in practice.

American Journal of Medical Quality, 2013, 28(1), 6–7. https://journals.sagepub.com/doi/full/10.1177/1062860612464731

6.24   Empathy in Medical Education and Patient Care

Mohammadreza Hojat, Salvatore Mangione, Joseph S. Gonnella,
Thomas Nasca, J. Jon Veloski, and Gregory Kane

In this commentary to a study in which a difference was found in the measure of empathy (Balanced Emotional Empathy Scale) between medical students who planned to pursue core specialties (e.g., family medicine, pediatrics) compared to other students who planned to pursue non-core specialties (e.g., radiology, pathology) we indicated that the study results were consistent with our previous research findings that physicians affiliated with the Jefferson Health Care System who were practicing in "people-oriented" specialties (e.g., primary care, obstetrics and gynecology, emergency medicine, psychiatry) obtained a significantly higher average of scores on the Jefferson Scale of Empathy than their counterparts in "technology-oriented" specialties (e.g., anesthesiology, pathology, radiology, orthopedic surgery, urology, surgery, and surgical subspecialties). Results remained unchanged when we controlled for the effect of gender. These findings are also in line with our early report of an empirical study that those interested in "people-oriented" specialty tend to value interpersonal relationships (social values) more than their counterparts in "technology-oriented" specialties. Emphasis was placed on the longitudinal study as opposed to cross-sectional study in addressing the development of empathy in medical students.

Academic Medicine (Letter to the Editor), 2001, *76*, 669.
   This abstract was written by the book editors.

6.25   Relationships Between Scores of the Jefferson Scale of Physician Empathy (JSPE) and the Interpersonal Reactivity Index (IRI)

Mohammadreza Hojat, Salvatore Mangione, Gregory C. Kane,
and Joseph S. Gonnella

We designed this study to examine the relationships between scores of two measures of empathy. One was specifically developed for measuring empathy in patient care situations; the other was developed for the general population. We hypothesized that the overlap between scores of the two measures would be greater for their constructs that are more relevant to patient care. Study participants were 93 first-year internal medicine residents at Thomas Jefferson University Hospital in Philadelphia. We administered the Jefferson Scale of Physician Empathy (JSPE, specifically developed for administration to health professionals) and the Interpersonal Reactivity Index (IRI, developed for the general population). We found statistically significant correlations of moderate magnitudes between the total scores of the JSPE and IRI ($r = 0.45$, $p < 0.01$). Our research hypothesis was confirmed by observing higher correlations between those scales of the IRI that were relevant to patient care (e.g., empathic concern, perspective taking) and related factors of the JSPE (compassionate care, perspective taking) than other scales of the IRI that seemed less relevant to patient care (e.g., personal distress and fantasy). These findings provide further support for the validity of the JSPE. We concluded that physician empathy as measured by the JSPE and its underlying factors are distinct personal attributes that have a limited overlap with fantasy and no overlap with personal distress defined as dimensions of an empathy measure that was developed for the general population.

Medical Teacher, 2005, *27*(7), 625–628. https://www.tandfonline.com/doi/full/10.1080/01421590500069744

6.26   The Jefferson Scale of Physician Empathy: Development and Preliminary Psychometric Data

Mohammadreza Hojat, Salvatore Mangione, Thomas J. Nasca,
Mitchell J. M. Cohen, Joseph S. Gonnella, James B. Erdmann, J. Jon Veloski,
and Mike Magee

Despite the importance of empathy in patient care, empirical investigation on the topic is scarce because there is no psychometrically sound instrument to operationally measure empathy in healthcare providers. This study was designed to develop a brief instrument to measure empathy in healthcare providers in patient care situations. Three groups participated in the study. Group 1 consisted of 55 physicians, Group 2 included 41 internal medicine residents, and Group 3 was comprised of 193 third-year medical students. A 90-item preliminary version of the empathy scale was developed based on a review of the literature and distributed to Group 1 for feedback. After pilot testing, a revised and shortened 45-item version of the instrument was distributed to Groups 2 and 3. Also included was a set of tests to measure other conceptually related attributes (e.g., compassion, concern, perspective taking, sympathy, warmth, dutifulness, faith in people). A final version of the Jefferson Scale of Physician Empathy containing 20 items based on statistical analyses was constructed. Psychometric findings provided support for construct validity, criterion-related validity (convergent and discriminant), and internal consistency reliability (coefficient alpha) of the scale. Suggestions are made for further research.

Educational and Psychological Measurement, 2001, *61*(2), 349–365.

6.27   An Empirical Study of Decline in Empathy in Medical School

Mohammadreza Hojat, Salvatore Mangione, Thomas J. Nasca,
Susan L. Rattner, James B. Erdmann, Joseph S. Gonnella, and Mike Magee

Context: It has been reported that students become more cynical as they progress through medical school. This can lead to a decline in empathy. Empirical research to address this issue is scarce because the definition of empathy lacks clarity, and a tool to measure empathy specifically in medical students and doctors has been unavailable.

Objective: To examine changes in empathy among medical students as they progress through medical school.

Materials and Subjects: A newly developed scale (Jefferson Scale of Physician Empathy (JSPE), with 20 Likert-type items) was administered to 125 medical students at the beginning (pretest) and end (posttest) of year 3 of medical school. This scale was specifically developed for measuring empathy in patient care situations and has acceptable psychometric properties.

Methods: In this prospective longitudinal study, the changes in pretest/posttest empathy scores were examined by using t-test for repeated measure design; the effect size estimates were also calculated.

Results: Statistically significant declines were observed in 5 items ($p < 0.01$) and in the total scores of the JSPE ($p < 0.05$) between the two test administrations.

Conclusions: Although the decline in empathy was not clinically important for all of the statistically significant findings, the downward trend suggests that empathy could be amenable to change during medical school. Further research is needed to identify factors that contribute to changes in empathy and to examine whether targeted educational programs can help to retain, reinforce, and cultivate empathy among medical students for improving clinical outcomes.

Medical Education, 2004, *38*(9), 934–941. https://onlinelibrary.wiley.com/doi/10.1111/j.1365-2929.2004.01911.x

6.28   Attitudes Toward Physician-Nurse Collaboration: A Cross-cultural Study of Male and Female Physicians and Nurses in the USA and Mexico

Mohammadreza Hojat, Thomas J. Nasca , Mitchell J. M. Cohen, Sylvia K. Fields, Susan L. Rattner, Margaret Griffiths, David Ibarra, Adelina Alcorta-Gonzalez, Antonio Torres-Ruiz, Guadalupe Ibarra, and Alma Garcia

Background: Interprofessional collaboration between physicians and nurses, within and between cultures, can help contain cost and insure better patient outcomes. Attitude toward such a collaboration is a function of the roles prescribed in the culture and guides professional behavior.

Objectives: The purpose of the study was to test three research hypotheses concerning attitudes toward physician-nurse collaboration across genders, disciplines, and cultures.

Method: The Jefferson Scale of Attitudes Toward Physician-Nurse Collaboration was administered to 639 physicians and nurses in the USA ($n = 267$) and Mexico ($n = 372$). Attitude scores were compared by gender (men, women), discipline (physicians, nurses), and culture (USA, Mexico) by using a three-way factorial analysis of variance design.

Results: Findings confirmed the first research hypothesis by demonstrating that both physicians and nurses in the USA would express more positive attitudes toward physician-nurse collaboration than their counterparts in Mexico. The second research hypothesis, positing that nurses as compared to physicians in both countries would express more positive attitudes toward physician-nurse collaboration, was also supported. The third research hypothesis that female physicians would express more positive attitudes toward physician-nurse collaboration than their male counterparts was not confirmed.

Conclusions: Collaborative education for medical and nursing students, particularly in cultures with a hierarchal model of interprofessional relationship, is needed to promote positive attitudes toward complementary roles of physicians and nurses. Faculty preparation for collaboration is necessary in such cultures before implementing collaborative education.

Nursing Research, 2001, *50*(2), 123–128.

6.29   An Operational Measure of Physician Lifelong Learning: Its Development, Components, and Preliminary Psychometric Data

Mohammadreza Hojat, Thomas J. Nasca, James B. Erdmann,
Anthony J. Frisby, J. Jon Veloski, and Joseph S. Gonnella

Despite the emphasis placed on physicians' lifelong learning, no psychometrically sound instrument has been developed to provide an operational measure of the concept and its components among physicians. The authors designed this study to develop a tool for measuring physician lifelong learning, to identify its underlying components and to assess its psychometric properties. A 37-item questionnaire was developed, based on a review of literature and the results of two pilot studies. Psychometric analyses of the responses of 160 physicians identified 19 items that were included in the Jefferson Scale of Physician Lifelong Learning. Factor analysis of the 19 items showed five meaningful factors that were consistent with the definition and major features of lifelong learning. They were "need recognition," "research endeavor," "self-initiation," "technical skills," and "personal motivation." The method of contrasted groups provided evidence in support of the validity of the five factors. The factors' reliability was assessed by coefficient alpha. It is concluded that lifelong learning is a multifaceted concept, and its operational measure is feasible for evaluating different educational programs and for studying group differences among physicians.

Medical   Teacher,   2003,   *25*(4),   433–437.   https://www.tandfonline.com/doi/abs/10.1080/0142159031000137463

6.30   Psychometrics of the Scale of Attitudes Toward Physician-Pharmacist Collaboration: A Study with Medical Students

Mohammadreza Hojat, John Spandorfer, Gerald A. Isenberg, Michael J. Vergare, Reza Fassihi, and Joseph S. Gonnella

Background: Despite the emphasis placed on interdisciplinary education and interprofessional collaboration between physicians and pharmacologists, no psychometrically sound instrument is available to measure attitudes toward collaborative relationships.

Aim: This study was designed to examine psychometrics of an instrument for measuring attitudes toward physician-pharmacist collaborative relationships for administration to students in medical and pharmacy schools and to physicians and pharmacists.

Methods: The Scale of Attitudes Toward Physician-Pharmacist Collaboration was completed by 210 students at Jefferson Medical College. Factor analysis and correlational methods were used to examine psychometrics of the instrument.

Results: Consistent with the conceptual framework of interprofessional collaboration, three underlying constructs, namely "responsibility and accountability," "shared authority," and "interdisciplinary education," emerged from the factor analysis of the instrument providing support for its construct validity. The reliability coefficient alpha for the instrument was 0.90. The instrument's criterion-related validity coefficient with scores of a validated instrument (Jefferson Scale of Attitudes Toward Physician-Nurse Collaboration) was 0.70.

Conclusions: Findings provide support for the validity and reliability of the instrument for medical students. The instrument has the potential to be used for the evaluation of interdisciplinary education in medical and pharmacy schools, and for the evaluation of patient outcomes resulting from collaborative physician-pharmacist relationships.

Medical Teacher, 2012, *34*(12), e833–837. https://www.tandfonline.com/doi/full/10.3109/0142159X.2012.714877

6.31 Measurement and Correlates of Physicians' Lifelong Learning

Mohammadreza Hojat, J. Jon Veloski, and Joseph S. Gonnella

Purpose: To examine the psychometric properties and correlates of an instrument to measure physicians' orientation toward lifelong learning with attention to differences between full-time and academic clinicians.

Method: The authors mailed a survey in 2006 to a national sample of 5349 alumni of Jefferson Medical College who graduated between 1975 and 2000; 3195 (60%) responded. The respondents were classified as full-time clinicians ($n = 1127$) and academic clinicians ($n = 1612$). The other 456 respondents were involved in administration or research. The revised Jefferson Scale of Physician Lifelong Learning (JeffSPLL) was included in the survey. Factor analysis, regression analysis, and analysis of variance were used to examine the construct- and criterion-related validities of the scale.

Results: Factor analysis of the JeffSPLL items resulted in three factors designated as "learning beliefs and motivation," "attention to learning opportunities," and "skills in seeking information," which supported its construct validity. Alpha reliability coefficients were 0.85 and 0.86, and test-retest reliability coefficients were 0.72 and 0.77 for full-time clinicians and academic clinicians, respectively. For full-time clinicians and academic clinicians, scores on the JeffSPLL were significantly ($p < 0.01$) correlated with measures of learning motivation, professional accomplishments, career satisfaction, and commitment to lifelong learning, which supported the criterion-related validity of the scale.

Conclusions: The findings indicate that the JeffSPLL is a psychometrically sound instrument that measures physicians' orientation toward lifelong learning among full-time clinicians and academic clinicians. The instrument can be used to monitor educational programs, assess educational outcomes, and examine group differences.

Academic Medicine, 2009, *84*(8), 1066–1074. https://doi.org/10.1097/ACM.0b013e3181acf25f

6.32   Physician Lifelong Learning: Conceptualization, Measurement, and Correlates in Full-Time Clinicians and Academic Clinicians

Mohammadreza Hojat, J. Jon Veloski, and Joseph S. Gonnella

Empirical research on lifelong learning in medicine has been scarce because of the ambiguity associated with its definition, as well as the lack of a psychometrically sound instrument to measure it. In this chapter, which is an expansion of our previous research, we present a definition of lifelong learning in medicine and report the psychometrics and correlates of an instrument (Jefferson Scale of Physician Lifelong Learning, JeffSPLL) that we began to develop in 2001 to specifically measure orientation toward lifelong learning among physicians and medical students. We collected survey data from 3195 physicians who were classified into three groups: full-time clinicians ($n = 1127$), academic clinicians ($n = 1612$), and others ($n = 456$). The three underlying components of the JeffSPLL resulted from factor analysis including "learning beliefs and motivation," "attention to learning opportunities," and "skills in seeking information." These factors correspond to the key features of lifelong learning often described in the literature, thus providing support for the construct validity of the JeffSPLL. Significant correlations between the JeffSPLL scores and the criterion measures of commitment to lifelong learning, learning motivation, information-seeking skills, professional accomplishments, career satisfaction, and academic performance support the criterion-related validity of the JeffSPLL for both full-time clinicians and academic clinicians. The reliability coefficients (coefficient alpha and test-retest) of the JeffSPLL ranged from 0.72 to 0.86 in both groups of physicians. In another study, the JeffSPLL was adapted for administration to medical students with satisfactory psychometric support. Implications of the findings in monitoring the outcomes of medical educational programs, and investigating differences across academic medical centers and groups of medical students and physicians, are discussed.

In M.P. Caltone (Ed). (2010), *Handbook of lifelong learning development* (pp. 37–78). New York: Nova Science Publishers.
    Reprinted with minor modifications in: Hojat, M., Veloski, J.J., & Gonnella, J. S. (2012). Physician lifelong learning: Conceptualization, measurement, and correlates in full-time clinicians, academic clinicians, and medical students. In *Continuing Professional Development and Lifelong Learning: Issues, Impacts and Outcomes*. Neimeyer, G.J. & Taylor, J.M., Nova Science Publishers (pp. 29–70).
    This abstract was written by the book editors.

6.33   Assessing Physicians' Orientation Toward Lifelong Learning

Mohammadreza Hojat, Jon Veloski, Thomas Nasca, James B. Erdmann,
and Joseph S. Gonnella

Background: Despite the importance of lifelong learning as an element of professionalism, no psychometrically sound instrument is available for its assessment among physicians.

Objective: To assess the validity and reliability of an instrument developed to measure physicians' orientation toward lifelong learning.

Design: Mail survey.

Participants: Seven hundred and twenty-one physicians, of whom 444 (62%) responded.

Measurement: The Jefferson Scale of Physician Lifelong Learning (JSPLL), which includes 19 items answered on a 4-point Likert scale, was used with additional questions about respondents' professional activities related to continuous learning.

Results: Factor analysis of the JSPLL yielded four subscales entitled "professional learning beliefs and motivation," "scholarly activities," "attention to learning opportunities," and "technical skills in seeking information," which are consistent with widely recognized features of lifelong learning. The validity of the scale and its subscales was supported by significant correlations with a set of criterion measures that presumably require continuous learning. The internal consistency reliability (coefficient α) of the JSPLL was 0.89, and the test-retest reliability was 0.91.

Conclusions: Empirical evidence supports the validity and reliability of the JSPLL.

Journal of General Internal Medicine, 2006, *21*(9), 931–936.

6.34   The Jefferson Scale of Attitudes Toward Interprofessional Collaboration (JEFFSATIC): Development and Multi-institution Psychometric Data

Mohammadreza Hojat, Julia Ward, John Spandorfer, Christine Arenson, Lon J. Van Winkle, and Brett Williams

This study was designed to develop a psychometrically sound instrument to measure attitudes toward interprofessional collaboration in health professions students and practitioners regardless of their professions and areas of practice. Based on a review of the literature a list of 27 items was generated, 12 faculty judged the face validity of the items, and 124 health profession faculty examined the content validity of the items. The preliminary version of the instrument was administered to 1976 health profession students in three universities (Thomas Jefferson University, $n = 510$; Midwestern University, $n = 392$; and Monash University, $n = 1074$). Twenty items that survived the psychometric scrutiny were included in the Jefferson Scale of Attitudes Toward Interprofessional Collaboration (JeffSATIC). Two constructs of "working relationships" and "accountability" emerged from factor analysis of the JeffSATIC. Cronbach's α coefficients for the JeffSATIC ranged from 0.84 to 0.90 in the three samples. Women obtained significantly higher JeffSATIC mean scores than men. Medical students obtained lower mean score on the JeffSATIC than most other health professions students at the same university. Psychometric support from a relatively large sample size of students in a variety of health profession programs in this multi-institutional study is encouraging which adds to the credibility of the JeffSATIC.

Journal of Interprofessional Care, 2015, 29, 238–244. https://www.tandfonline.com/doi/full/10.3109/13561820.2014.962129

6.35   Empathy in Medical Students as Related to Specialty Interest, Personality, and Perceptions of Mother and Father

Mohammadreza Hojat, Marvin Zuckerman, Joseph S. Gonnella,
Salvatore Mangione, Thomas J. Nasca, Michael J. Vergare, and Mike Magee

This study was designed to examine relationships between empathy, specialty interest, personality, and perceptions of mother and father. Participants were 422 first-year medical students who completed the Jefferson Scale of Physician Empathy (JSPE) and the Zuckerman-Kuhlman Personality Questionnaire (ZKPQ, short form). They also reported their specialty interest and their perceptions of early relationships with their parents. Results showed that women outscored men on the empathy scale. Also, we found that higher scores on the JSPE were associated with students' interest in people-oriented specialties (as opposed to procedure- and technology-oriented specialties), higher level of satisfaction with early maternal relationship, higher sociability, and lower aggressive-hostility scores. Controlling for gender and social desirability did not change the general pattern of findings.

Personality and Individual Differences, 2005, *39*(7), 1205–1215.
    Reprinted with permission from Elsevier.

6.36 Enhancing Student Empathetic Engagement, History-Taking, and Communication Skills During Electronic Medical Record Use in Patient Care

Alisa Alfonsi Lo Sasso, Courtney E. Lamberton, Mary Sammon, Katherine T. Berg, John W. Caruso, Jonathan Cass, and Mohammadreza Hojat

Purpose: To examine whether an intervention on proper use of electronic medical records (EMRs) in patient care could help improve medical students' empathic engagement, and to test the hypothesis that the training would reduce communication hurdles in clinical encounters.

Method: Seventy third-year medical students from the Sidney Kimmel Medical College at Thomas Jefferson University were randomly divided into intervention and control groups during their 6-week pediatric clerkship in 2012–2013. The intervention group received a 1-h training session on EMR-specific communication skills, including discussion of EMR use, the SALTED mnemonic and technique (Set-up, Ask, Listen, Type, Exceptions, Documentation), and role-plays. Both groups completed the Jefferson Scale of Empathy (JSE) at the clerkship's start and end. At clerkship's end, faculty and standardized patients (SPs) rated students' empathic engagement in SP encounters, using the Jefferson Scale of Patient Perceptions of Physician Empathy (JSPPPE), and their history-taking and communication skills.

Results: Faculty mean ratings on the JSPPPE, history-taking skills, and communication skills were significantly higher for the intervention group than the control group. SP mean ratings on history-taking skills were significantly higher for the intervention group than the control group. Both groups' JSE mean scores increased pretest to posttest, but the changes were not significant. The intervention group's posttest JSE mean score was higher than the control group's, but the difference was not significant.

Conclusions: The findings suggest that a simple intervention providing specialized training in EMR-specific communication can improve medical students' empathic engagement in patient care, history-taking skills, and communication skills.

Academic Medicine, 2017, *92*(7), 1022–1027. https://doi.org/10.1097/ACM.0000000000001476

6.37   Assessment of Empathy in Different Years of Internal Medicine Training

Salvatore Mangione, Gregory C. Kane, John W. Caruso, Joseph S. Gonnella, Thomas J. Nasca, and Mohammadreza Hojat

Problem Statement and Background: The issue of operational measurement of physician empathy and the question of whether empathy could change at different levels of medical education are of interest to medical educators.

Methods: We studied 98 internal medicine residents from all 3 years of training. We administered the Jefferson Scale of Physician Empathy and correlated residents' empathy scores with ratings on humanistic attributes by program directors.

Results: There were no statistically significant differences in empathy scores among residents of different training levels. Empathy scores remained also stable during one year of internship (test-retest reliability = 0.72). Correlation between empathy and ratings on humanism was 0.17.

Conclusions: Findings suggest that empathy is a relatively stable trait that is not easily amendable to change in residency training program. The issue of whether targeted educational activities for the purpose of cultivating empathy can improve the empathy scores awaits empirical scrutiny.

Medical Teacher, 2002, 24(4), 370–373. https://www.tandfonline.com/doi/abs/10.1080/01421590220145725

6.38   Evaluating the Relationship Between Participation in Student-Run Free Clinics and Changes in Empathy in Medical Students

Anita Modi, Michele Fascelli, Zachary Daitch, and Mohammadreza Hojat

Purpose: We explored differences in changes in medical student empathy in the third year of medical school between volunteers at JeffHOPE, a multisite medical student-run free clinic of Sidney Kimmel Medical College (SKMC), and non-volunteers.

Method: Volunteerism and leadership experience at JeffHOPE were documented for medical students in the class of 2015 ($n = 272$) across their medical educations. Students completed the Jefferson Scale of Empathy at the beginning of medical school and at the end of the third year. Students who reported participation in other Jefferson-affiliated clinics ($n = 44$) were excluded from this study. Complete data were available for 188 SKMC students.

Results: Forty-five percent of students ($n = 85$) volunteered at JeffHOPE at least once during their medical educations. Fifteen percent of students ($n = 48$) were selected for leadership positions involving weekly clinic participation. Non-volunteers demonstrated significant decline in empathy in medical school ($p = 0.009$), while those who volunteered at JeffHOPE at least once over the course of their medical education did not show any significant decline ($p = 0.07$).

Conclusions: These findings suggest that medical students may benefit from volunteering at student-run free clinics to care for underserved populations throughout medical school.

Journal of Primary Care & Community Health, 2017, *8*(3), 122–126.

Copyright© 2017. Sage Publishing. https://journals.sagepub.com/doi/10.1177/2150131916685199

6.39   Measuring Professionalism: A Review of Studies with Instruments Reported in the Literature Between 1982 and 2002

J. Jon Veloski, Sylvia K. Fields, James R. Boex, and Linda L. Blank

Purpose: To describe the measurement properties of instruments reported in the literature that faculty might use to measure professionalism in medical students and residents.

Method: The authors reviewed studies published between 1982 and 2002 that had been located using Medline and four other databases. A national panel of 12 experts in measurement and research in medical education extracted data from research reports using a structured critique form.

Results: A total of 134 empirical studies related to the concept of professionalism were identified. The content of 114 involved specific elements of professionalism such as ethics, humanism, and multiculturalism, or associated phenomena in the educational environment such as abuse and cheating. Few studies addressed professionalism as a comprehensive construct (11 studies) or as a distinct facet of clinical competence (9 studies). The purpose of 109 studies was research or program evaluation rather than summative or formative assessment. Sixty-five used self-administered instruments with no independent observation of the participants' professional behavior. Evidence of reliability was reported in 62 studies. Although content validity was reported in 86 studies, only 34 provided strong evidence. Evidence of concurrent or predictive validity was provided in 43 and 16 studies, respectively.

Conclusions: There are few well-documented studies of instruments that can be used to measure professionalism in formative or summative evaluation. When evaluating the tools described in published research, it is essential for faculty to look critically for evidence related to the three fundamental measurement properties of content validity, reliability, and practicality.

Academic Medicine, 2005, *80*(4), 366–370. https://journals.lww.com/academic-medicine/Fulltext/2005/04000/Measuring_Professionalism_A_Review_of_Studies.14.aspx

6.40   Linguistic Analysis of Empathy in Medical School Admission Essays

Mary E. Yaden, David B. Yaden, Anneke E. K. Buffone, Johannes C. Eichstaedt, Patrick Crutchley, Laura K. Smith, Jonathan L. Cass, Clara A. Callahan, Susan R. Rosenthal, Lyle H. Ungar, Andrew Schwartz, and Mohammadreza Hojat

Objectives: This study aimed to determine whether words used in medical school admission essays can predict physician empathy.

Methods: A computational form of linguistic analysis was used for the content analysis of medical school admission essays. Words in medical school admission essays were computationally grouped into 20 "topics" which were then correlated with scores on the Jefferson Scale of Empathy. The study sample included 1805 matriculants (between 2008 and 2015) at a single medical college in the North East of the USA who wrote an admission essay and completed the Jefferson Scale of Empathy at matriculation.

Results: After correcting for multiple comparisons and controlling for gender, the Jefferson Scale of Empathy scores significantly correlated with a linguistic topic ($r = 0.074$, $p < 0.05$). This topic comprised of specific words used in essays such as "understanding," "compassion," "empathy," "feeling," and "trust." These words are related to themes emphasized in both theoretical writing and empirical studies on physician empathy.

Conclusions: This study demonstrates that physician empathy can be predicted from medical school admission essays. The implications of this methodological capability, i.e., to quantitatively associate linguistic features or words with psychometric outcomes, bear on the future of medical education research and admission. In particular, these findings suggest that those responsible for medical school admissions could identify more empathetic applicants based on the language of their application essays.

International Journal of Medical Education, 2020, *11*, 186–190. https://www.ijme. net/archive/11/linguistic-analysis-of-empathy/

Chapter 7
Miscellaneous

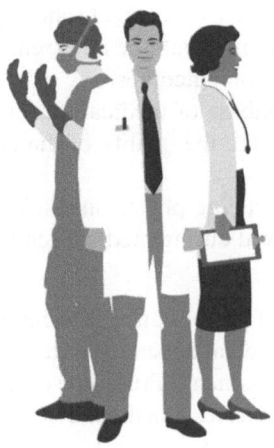

Contents

7.1 Medical Education, Social Accountability, and Patient Outcomes........................ 225
7.2 AM Last Page: The Jefferson Longitudinal Study of Medical Education................ 226
7.3 Viewpoint: Guiding Medical Students Toward Empathetic Patient Care................ 228
7.4 Jefferson Medical College Longitudinal Study: A Prototype for Evaluation
    of Changes... 229
7.5 Creating a Longitudinal Database in Medical Education: Perspectives
    from the Pioneers... 230
7.6 Disciplinary Action by Medical Boards and Prior Behavior in Medical School......... 231
7.7 The Jefferson Longitudinal Study of Medical Education: Five Decades
    of Outcome Assessment... 232

Abstract

- This chapter includes reported highlights of findings from publications that could not be classified in other sections.
- Medical schools should be responsible for collecting pertinent data with which to assess and monitor their educational programs and outcomes.
- Medical schools should develop a longitudinal study of medical education outcomes and use psychometrically sound instruments to assess achievement of their educational goals.
- Longitudinal study of medical students and graduates is a core mandate of every medical school.

- The Jefferson project on physician empathy generally confirmed that empathy in patient care must be considered as an important component of physician's overall competence and is a significant factor in optimal patient outcomes.
- Assessments of clinical competence of medical school graduates in the first year of postgraduate medical education should be an essential component of a longitudinal study of medical education outcomes.
- Establishing a longitudinal database of medical students and graduates enables medical schools to test and ensure the quality of the doctors they produce, and justifies curricular reforms.
- Disciplinary action against practicing physicians is found to be associated with unprofessional behavior observed during medical school.

Keywords Content and context of performance · Disciplinary action · Insurance and governmental regulations · Medical education outcomes · Pertinent personal qualities · PGY1 performance assessment · Prototype of assessment · Social accountability · Ultimate goal · Unprofessional behavior

7.1   Medical Education, Social Accountability, and Patient Outcomes

Joseph S. Gonnella and Mohammadreza Hojat

Medicine is a public service profession; thus, social accountability is an integral feature of medical education and practice of medicine. The ultimate goal of medical education is to improve patient outcomes including physical, mental, and social well-being of the patient. From a broad perspective, physician performance to achieve optimal patient outcomes is a function of two basic components: *content* and *context*. The content component includes physician's characteristics such as medical knowledge, clinical and procedural skills, and personal qualities. Social accountability obligates medical education to ensure that physicians in training have acquired sufficient knowledge, developed adequate clinical skills, and cultivated pertinent personal qualities in order to guarantee public safety. The contextual component accounts for other factors that are often beyond the physician's control, but either directly or indirectly influence patient outcomes, such as the disease severity, insurance and governmental regulations, biotechnical availability, collaboration of other health professionals, and the patient's culture and reward systems. Social accountability in medical education calls for preparing physicians in training to handle the aforementioned contextual issues. Medical schools should be held responsible for collecting pertinent data with which to assess and monitor their educational programs and outcomes. For that purpose, medical schools must be required to develop longitudinal study of medical education outcomes and use psychometrically sound instruments to assess the extent to which their educational goals have been achieved. To honor the principle of social accountability, assessments of educational outcomes should be mandatory for all medical schools. Thus, documenting the achievement of educational goals should be seen as a core mandate of every medical school, rather than as a luxury held by only a few.

Medical Education, 2012, *46*(1), 3–4. https://onlinelibrary.wiley.com/doi/ 10.1111/j.1365-2923.2011.04157.x

7.2 AM Last Page: The Jefferson Longitudinal Study of Medical Education

Joseph S. Gonnella, Mohammadreza Hojat, and J. Jon Veloski

We prepared a snapshot of the Jefferson Longitudinal Study (JLS) in response to an invitation from Academic Medicine to prepare a one-page schematic summary of the JLS for publication in the journal. The JLS is the most comprehensive, extensive, and uninterrupted tracking system of medical students of its kind maintained in a single medical school. The study was initiated in 1970 based on the premise that medical schools have an obligation to society to monitor their educational outcomes. The intention was to track every medical student who entered Jefferson (currently Sidney Kimmel) Medical College throughout medical school, postgraduate education, and professional career. Data for the JLS are routinely updated starting from entering class of 1964 to the present time using information from the Association of American Medical Colleges, American Medical Association, American Board of Medical Specialties, National Board of Medical Examiners, in-house sources, and surveys. The major goals of the JLS include service and research. Service is often provided to academic committees (e.g., providing data to assess admission trends and policies); college/dean's office/administrators (e.g., providing data for the annual report, dean's letters of evaluations, providing supporting data for accreditation); faculty (e.g., responding to their inquiries); and student (guiding academic and career development). Also, JLS serves as a source to empirically address issues of interest to college's senior administrators, faculty, and students. In addition, data have been retrieved from the database of the JLS to address issues of interest to leaders in medical education and medical education communities through publication in peer-reviewed journals and presentations in national and international meetings. The JLS data include information prior to medical school (e.g., demographics, SAT and MCAT scores, undergraduate GPAs in science and nonscience courses); performance during medical school (e.g., course evaluations and examination grades, clerkship competence ratings, and information from a matriculation survey that is administered at first-year orientation session on students' personal qualities including empathic orientation toward patient care, attitudes, and plans, and from an exit survey that is administered in the last year of medical school during residency match result session on students' assessments of academic programs and future plans); and results of medical licensing examinations (USMLE Steps 1, 2, 3, NBME Parts 1, 2, 3). In addition, after-medical school and career data (e.g., specialty, subspecialty choices, postgraduate training institutions, geographical locations of residency training and practice, board certification status, faculty appointment type of practice, active status, and occasional follow-up surveys) are also maintained in the JLS. One unique feature of the JLS is the ratings of graduates' clinical competence made at the completion of the first residency year by residency program directors for those graduates who grant us permission for collecting such data. Some of our new psychometrically sound instruments developed for the assessments of educational and patient outcomes are also described in this snapshot of the JLS.

Academic Medicine, 2011, *86*(3), 404.

https://journals.lww.com/academicmedicine/fulltext/2011/03000/am_last_page__the_jefferson_longitudinal_study_of.34.aspx

7.3 Viewpoint: Guiding Medical Students Toward Empathetic Patient Care

Mohammadreza Hojat

In response to a request from the AAMC Reporter on the viewpoint of the author of the Jefferson Scale of Empathy (JSE) about Jefferson empathy research in medical students, Dr. Hojat indicated that empathic engagement is the pillar of the patient-physician relationship that is beneficial not only to the patient, but also to the physician. The basic human need to be understood is fulfilled through an empathic relationship that lays the foundation for a trusting relationship leading to greater compliance, and thus more optimal patient outcomes. Our empirical research by retrieving data from the Jefferson Longitudinal Study showed that medical students' higher scores on the JSE were significantly associated with higher faculty ratings of clinical competence in core clerkships, simulated patients' assessments of students' empathic engagement in Objective Structured Clinical Examinations, peer nominations on professionalism attributes, attitudes toward interprofessional collaboration, and interest in pursuing people-oriented specialties (e.g., primary care) as opposed to technology/procedure-oriented specialties (e.g., hospital-based specialties such as pathology, anesthesiology, radiology). These findings suggest that empathy in patient care must be placed in the realm of evidence-based medicine. We have also found that empathy tends to erode in the third year of medical school when the curriculum shifts from preclinical to clinical phase of medical education, ironically when empathy is most needed. Our research indicates that empathy can be enhanced in medical students by their participation in targeted educational programs; however, increase in empathic orientation toward patient showed only a short-term effect, and thus could not be sustained for a long time unless reinforced by additional educational remedies. We have also shown that physicians' scores on the JSE were significantly associated with patient outcomes in diabetic patients (indicated by results of laboratory tests such as A1C and LDL-C). Our findings generally suggest that empathy must be considered as an important component of physician's overall competence and a significant factor in optimal patient outcomes. More research is needed to identify factors that erode medical students' empathy, and to explore more effective approaches to enhance and sustain empathy. The future research agenda gets longer rather than shorter with new findings, raising more questions than answers in our embarking journey in this uncharted territory.

AAMC Reporter, 2012, *21*(6), 3.
    This abstract was written by the book editors.

7.4   Jefferson Medical College Longitudinal Study: A Prototype for Evaluation of Changes

Mohammadreza Hojat, Joseph S. Gonnella, J. Jon Veloski, and James B. Erdmann

Assessment of medical education outcomes and effect of changes on medical education curriculum must be based on empirical data rather than anecdotal observations. Such evaluations call for a longitudinal study design to examine changes from the beginning of medical education and throughout postgraduate medical education and professional career. To provide information for the development of such a study, the history, scope, goals, and sample of outcome research of the Jefferson Longitudinal Study are briefly described, and required resources for the development and maintenance of such a longitudinal study are outlined. The Jefferson Longitudinal Study demonstrates that a longitudinal study of medical education outcomes provides a unique opportunity to collect pertinent data for monitoring educational programs and for systematic empirical assessment of educational outcomes. The interest in the Jefferson Longitudinal Study expressed by other medical schools, viewing this study as a prototypical model for medical education outcome assessment, suggests that such a longitudinal study should be seen as a core mandate for every medical school.

Education for Health, 1996, *9*, 99–113.
This abstract was written by the book editors.

7.5   Creating a Longitudinal Database in Medical Education: Perspectives from the Pioneers

Rashmi A. Kusurkar and Gerda Croiset

The Jefferson Longitudinal Study of Medical Education (JLSME) is the longest running database in medical education and covers the collection and measurement of background, learning, performance, and psychosocial variables before, during, and after medical school. Recently, our research group at VU University Medical Center School of Medical Sciences launched a longitudinal study in medical education, called the "Student Motivation and Success Study." While setting up this study, we faced many challenges and learning about the JLSME helped us gain a fresh perspective on our work. We interviewed Drs. Joseph Gonnella and Mohammadreza Hojat, the leaders of the JLSME, and present their experiences verbatim in this study and summarize the lessons we learned as tips for others. We conclude that by establishing a longitudinal database, medical educators can test and ensure the quality of the doctors they produce, justify curricular reforms, participate in a continuing inquiry into their educational practices, and produce more generalizable research findings.

Education for Health, 2016, *29*, 266–270. https://www.educationforhealth.net/article.asp?issn=1357-6283;year=2016;volume=29;issue=3;spage=266;epage=270;au last=Kusurkar

This abstract was written by the book editors.

7.6   Disciplinary Action by Medical Boards and Prior Behavior in Medical School

Maxine A. Papadakis, Arianne Teherani, Mary A. Banach, Timothy R. Knettler, Susan L. Rattner, David T. Stern, J. Jon Veloski, and Carol S. Hodgson

Background: Evidence supporting professionalism as a critical measure of competence in medical education is limited. In this case–control study, we investigated the association of disciplinary action against practicing physicians with prior unprofessional behavior in medical school. We also examined the specific types of behavior that are most predictive of disciplinary action against practicing physicians with unprofessional behavior in medical school.

Methods: The study included 235 graduates of three medical schools who were disciplined by one of 40 state medical boards between 1990 and 2003 (case physicians). The 469 control physicians were matched with the case physicians according to medical school and graduation year. Predictor variables from medical school included the presence or absence of narratives describing unprofessional behavior, grades, standardized test scores, and demographic characteristics. Narratives were assigned an overall rating for unprofessional behavior. Those that met the threshold for unprofessional behavior were further classified among eight types of behavior and assigned a severity rating (moderate to severe).

Results: Disciplinary action by a medical board was strongly associated with prior unprofessional behavior in medical school (odds ratio, 3.0; 95% confidence interval, 1.9–4.8), for a population attributable risk of disciplinary action of 26%. The types of unprofessional behavior most strongly linked with disciplinary action were severe irresponsibility (odds ratio, 8.5; 95% confidence interval, 1.8–40.1) and severely diminished capacity for self-improvement (odds ratio, 3.1; 95% confidence interval, 1.2–8.2). Disciplinary action by a medical board was also associated with low scores on the Medical College Admission Test and poor grades in the first 2 years of medical school (1% and 7% population attributable risk, respectively), but the association with these variables was less strong than that with unprofessional behavior.

Conclusions: In this case–control study, disciplinary action among practicing physicians by medical boards was strongly associated with unprofessional behavior in medical schools. Students with the strongest association were those who were described as irresponsible or as having diminished ability to improve their behavior. Professionalism should have a central role in medical academics and throughout one's medical career.

The New England Journal of Medicine, 2005, *353*(25), 2673–2682.

7.7   The Jefferson Longitudinal Study of Medical Education: Five Decades of Outcome Assessment

J. Jon Veloski, Mohammadreza Hojat, and Joseph S. Gonnella

This study marks five decades of continuity of the Jefferson Longitudinal Study of Medical Education. Conceived upon a belief that medical schools have a professional and social obligation to monitor the quality of their educational outcomes, the Jefferson Longitudinal Study has served for five decades as a source to monitor educational programs, professionalism progress, and academic management, and also served as a resource for faculty development and institutional research. In addition, data retrieved from the JLS database, which comprises millions of pieces of data points, have produced a large number of publications in peer-reviewed journals empirically addressing questions raised by academic medical leaders, medical education researchers, and medical school faculty. The Jefferson Longitudinal Study has established a leadership role in monitoring important professional career outcomes not routinely tracked by professional organizations. For example, new psychometrically sound instruments have been developed to measure aspects of professional development, such as orientation toward lifelong learning, interprofessional collaboration and teamwork, and empathic orientation toward patient care in physicians in training and in practice. In addition, the Jefferson Longitudinal Study provides systematic and uninterrupted empirical information on cohorts of medical students throughout medical school, residency, and professional life to assess short- and long-term outcomes of admission policies, special programs, curriculum innovations, and complex issues in students' academic progress and professional development. Throughout the graduate's career, the Jefferson Longitudinal Study tracks key professional outcomes, which are continuously monitored and updated such as faculty appointments, board certification status, employment and practice setting changes, and geographical location of practice. The Jefferson Longitudinal Study provides a solid foundation of institutional research on educational and professional outcomes, enabling the faculty and administration to assess the extent to which the program goals have been achieved, and also providing pertinent information required by accreditation bodies such as the Liaison Committee on Medical Education (LCME) and the Middle States Commission on Higher Education.

Population Health Matters (Formerly Health Policy Newsletter), 2013, *26*(1), 2–3.
    This abstract was written by the book editors.

Bibliography

Ashikawa, H., Hojat, M., Zeleznik, C., & Gonnella, J. S. (1991). Reexamination of relationships between students' undergraduate majors, medical school performances, and career plans at Jefferson Medical College. *Academic Medicine, 66*, 458–464. https://doi.org/10.1097/00001888-199108000-00009 [13][1].

Ashikawa, H., Xu, G., & Veloski, J. J. (1992). Students' ratings of otolaryngology clerkship activities: The role of residents. *Medical Teacher, 14*, 77–81. https://doi.org/10.3109/01421599209044019 [54].

Berg, K., Blatt, B., Lopreiato, J., Jung, J., Schaeffer, A., Heil, D., Owens, T., Carter-Nolan, P. L., Berg, D., Veloski, J., Darby, E., & Hojat, M. (2015). Standardized patient assessment of medical student empathy: Ethnicity and gender effects in a multi-institutional study. *Academic Medicine, 90*(1), 105–111. https://doi.org/10.1097/ACM.0000000000000529 [30].

Berg, K., Majdan, J. F., Berg, D., Veloski, J., & Hojat, M. (2011a). A comparison of medical students' self-reported empathy with simulated patients' assessments of the students' empathy. *Medical Teacher, 33*(5), 388–391. https://doi.org/10.3109/0142159X.2010.530319 [55].

Berg, K., Majdan, J. F., Berg, D., Veloski, J., & Hojat, M. (2011b). Medical students' self-reported empathy and simulated patients' assessments of student empathy: An analysis by gender and ethnicity. *Academic Medicine, 86*, 984–988. https://doi.org/10.1097/ACM.0b013e3182224f1f [182].

Berg, K., Winward, M., Clauser, B. E., Veloski, J. A., Berg, D., Dillon, G. F., & Veloski, J. J. (2008). The relationship between performance on a medical school's clinical skills assessment and USMLE Step 2 CS. *Academic Medicine, 83*(10), S37–S40. https://doi.org/10.1097/ACM.0b013e318183cb5c [56].

Blacklow, R. S., Goepp, C. E., & Hojat, M. (1991). Class ranking models for Deans' letters and their psychometric evaluation. *Academic Medicine, 66*, S10–S12. https://doi.org/10.1097/00001888-199109000-00025 [79].

Blacklow, R. S., Goepp, C. E., & Hojat, M. (1993). Further psychometric evaluations of a class ranking model as a predictor of graduates' clinical competence in the first year of residency. *Academic Medicine, 68*, 295–297. https://doi.org/10.1097/00001888-199304000-00017 [80].

Boulis, A., Jacobs, J., & Veloski, J. J. (2001). Gender segregation by specialty during medical school. *Academic Medicine, 76*, S65–S67. https://doi.org/10.1097/00001888-200110001-00022 [31].

Bu, P., Veloski, J. J., & Ankam, N. S. (2016). Effects of a brief curricular intervention on medical students' attitudes toward people with disabilities in healthcare settings. *American*

---

[1] The page number of the abstract in the document is shown in brackets.

Journal of Physical Medicine & Rehabilitation, 95(12), 939–945. https://doi.org/10.1097/PHM.0000000000000535 [137].

Bucher, J. T., Vu, D. M., & Hojat, M. (2013). Psychostimulant drug abuse and personality factors in medical students. *Medical Teacher, 35*(1), 53–57. https://doi.org/10.3109/0142159X.2012.731099 [138].

Callahan, C. A., Erdmann, J. B., Hojat, M., Veloski, J. J., Rattner, S. L., Nasca, T. J., & Gonnella, J. S. (2000). Validity of faculty ratings of students' clinical competence in core clerkships in relation to scores on licensing examinations and supervisors' ratings in residency. *Academic Medicine, 75*(Supplement), 71–73. https://doi.org/10.1097/00001888-200010001-00023 [57].

Callahan, C. A., Hojat, M., & Gonnella, J. S. (2007). Volunteer bias in medical education research: An empirical study of over three decades of longitudinal data. *Medical Education, 41*(8), 746–753. https://doi.org/10.1111/j.1365-2923.2007.02803.x [139].

Callahan, C. A., Hojat, M., Veloski, J., Erdmann, J. B., & Gonnella, J. S. (2010). The predictive validity of three versions of the MCAT in relation to performance in medical school, residency, and licensing examinations: A longitudinal study of 36 classes of Jefferson Medical College. *Academic Medicine, 85*(6), 980–987. https://doi.org/10.1097/ACM.0b013e3181cece3d [4].

Callahan, C. A., Veloski, J. J., Xu, G., Hojat, M., Zeleznik, C., & Gonnella, J. S. (1992). The Jefferson-Penn State B.S.-M.D. program: A 26-year experience. *Academic Medicine, 67*, 792–797. https://doi.org/10.1097/00001888-199211000-00019 [14].

Collier, V. U., Hojat, M., Rattner, S. L., Gonnella, J. S., Erdmann, J. B., Nasca, T. J., & Veloski, J. J. (2001). Correlates of young physicians' support for unionization to maintain professional influence. *Academic Medicine, 76*, 1039–1044. https://doi.org/10.1097/00001888-200110000-00014 [96].

Cooter, R., Erdmann, J. B., Gonnella, J. S., Callahan, C. A., Hojat, M., & Xu, G. (2004). Economic diversity in medical education: The relationship between students' family income and academic performance, career choice, and student debt. *Evaluation & the Health Professions, 27*, 252–264. https://doi.org/10.1177/0163278704267041 [140].

Erdmann, J. B., Hojat, M., & Veloski, J. J. (1992). Comparing the accuracies of entire-group and subgroup models to predict NBME-I scores for medical school applicants. *Academic Medicine, 67*, 860–862. https://doi.org/10.1097/00001888-199212000-00014 [32].

Fenderson, B. A., Hojat, M., Damjanov, I., & Rubin, E. (1999). Characteristics of medical students completing an honors program in pathology. *Human Pathology, 30*, 1296–1301. https://doi.org/10.1016/S0046-8177(99)90059-X [141].

Fields, S. K., Hojat, M., Gonnella, J. S., Mangione, S., Kane, G. C., & Magee, M. (2004). Comparisons of nurses and physicians on an operational measure of empathy. *Evaluation & the Health Professions, 27*, 80–94. https://doi.org/10.1177/0163278703261206 [183].

Forouzan, I., & Hojat, M. (1993). Stability and change of interest in obstetrics-gynecology among medical students: Eighteen years of longitudinal data. *Academic Medicine, 68*, 919–222. https://doi.org/10.1097/00001888-199312000-00013 [97].

Gartland, J., Hojat, M., Christian, E. B., Callahan, C. A., & Nasca, T. J. (2003). African American and white physicians: A comparison of satisfaction with medical education, professional careers and research activities. *Teaching and Learning in Medicine, 15*, 106–112. https://doi.org/10.1207/S15328015TLM1502_06 [33].

Glaser, K., Hojat, M., & Callahan, C. A. (1996). Evaluation of an enrichment programme for entering medical students predicted to be in need of academic preparation. *Education for Health, 9*, 221–228. [15].

Glaser, K., Hojat, M., Veloski, J. J., Blacklow, R. S., & Goepp, C. E. (1992). Science, verbal, or quantitative skills: Which is the most important predictor of physician competence? *Educational and Psychological Measurement, 52*, 395–406. https://journals.sagepub.com/doi/pdf/10.1177/0013164492052002015 [5].

Gonnella, J. S., Callahan, C. A., Erdmann, J. B., Veloski, J. J., Jafari, N., Markle, R. A., & Hojat, M. (2021). Preparing for the MD: How long, at what cost, and with what outcomes? *Academic Medicine, 96*, 101–107. https://doi.org/10.1097/ACM.0000000000003298 [16].

Gonnella, J. S., Callahan, C. A., Louis, D. Z., Hojat, M., & Erdmann, J. B. (2004a). Medical education and health services research: The linkage. *Medical Teacher, 26*, 7–11. https://doi.org/10.1080/0142159032000156515 [98].

Gonnella, J. S., Erdmann, J. B., & Hojat, M. (2004b). An empirical study of the predictive validity of number grades in medical school using 3 decades of longitudinal data: Implications for a grading system. *Medical Education, 38*, 425–434. https://doi.org/10.1111/j.1365-2923.2004.01774.x [50].

Gonnella, J. S., & Hojat, M. (1983). Relationship between performance in medical school and postgraduate competence. *Journal of Medical Education, 58*, 679–685. https://psycnet.apa.org/record/1984-15992-001 [81].

Gonnella, J. S., & Hojat, M. (2001). Biotechnology and ethics in medical education of the new millennium: Physician roles and responsibilities. *Medical Teacher, 23*, 371–377. https://doi.org/10.1080/01421590120042982 [142].

Gonnella, J. S., & Hojat, M. (2012). Medical education, social accountability and patient outcomes. *Medical Education, 46*(1), 3–4. https://doi.org/10.1111/j.1365-2923.2011.04157.x [225].

Gonnella, J. S., Hojat, M., Erdmann, J. B., & Veloski, J. J. (Eds.). (1993a). *Assessment measures in medical school, residency, and practice: The connections.* Springer. [84].

Gonnella, J. S., Hojat, M., Erdmann, J. B., & Veloski, J. J. (1993b). A case of mistaken identity: Signal and noise in connecting performance assessments before and after graduation from medical school. *Academic Medicine, 68*(Supplement), S9–S16. https://doi.org/10.1097/00001888-199302000-00023 [82].

Gonnella, J. S., Hojat, M., Erdmann, J. B., & Veloski, J. J. (1993c). What have we learned, and where do we go from here? *Academic Medicine, 68*(Supplement), S79–S87. https://doi.org/10.1097/00001888-199302000-00036 [83].

Gonnella, J. S., Hojat, M., Erdmann, J. B., & Veloski, J. J. (1996). The impact of early career specialization on licensing requirements and related educational implications. *Advances in Health Sciences Education, 1*, 125–139. https://doi.org/10.1007/BF00159277 [99].

Gonnella, J. S., Hojat, M., Erdmann, J. B., & Veloski, J. J. (1998). The role of resident performance evaluation in board certification. In E. L. Mancall & P. G. Bashook (Eds.), *Evaluating residents for board certification* (pp. 3–14). American Board of Medical Specialties. [85].

Gonnella, J. S., Hojat, M., & Veloski, J. J. (2011). AM last page: The Jefferson longitudinal study of medical education. *Academic Medicine, 86*(3), 404. https://doi.org/10.1097/ACM.0b013e31820bb3e7 [226].

Gonnella, J. S., Hojat, M., Veloski, J. J., & Zeleznik, C. (1983). Measuring the contribution of medical education to patient care: A review. *Proceedings of the Annual Conference on Research in Medical Education, 22*, 3–16. https://pubmed.ncbi.nlm.nih.gov/6564875/ [86].

Gonnella, J. S., & Veloski, J. J. (1982). The impact of early specialization on the clinical competence of residents. *The New England Journal of Medicine, 306*, 275–277. https://doi.org/10.1056/NEJM198202043060505 [100].

Gottlieb, J., Fields, S. K., Hojat, M., & Veloski, J. J. (1995). Should half of all medical school graduates enter primary care? Perceptions of faculty members at Jefferson Medical College. *Academic Medicine, 70*, 1125–1133. https://pubmed.ncbi.nlm.nih.gov/7495458/ [101].

Herman, M. W. (1984). Medical students' opinions concerning the healthcare system. *Journal of Community Health, 9*, 196–205. https://doi.org/10.1007/BF01326700 [144].

Herman, M. W. (1985). Medical students' opinions concerning the healthcare system. *Journal of Medical Education, 60*, 431–438. https://doi.org/10.1097/00001888-198506000-00001 [143].

Herman, M. W., & Veloski, J. J. (1977). Family medicine and primary care: Trends and student characteristics. *Journal of Medical Education, 52*, 99–106. https://doi.org/10.1097/00001888-197702000-00002 [102].

Herman, M. W., & Veloski, J. J. (1980). Performance and career expectations of women medical students: A comparison with men (Letter to the Editor). *The New England Journal of Medicine, 302*, 1035–1036. [34].

Herman, M. W., & Veloski, J. J. (1981). Premedical training, personal characteristics and performance in medical school. *Medical Education, 15*, 363–367. https://doi.org/10.1111/j.1365-2923.1981.tb02415.x [17].

Herman, M. W., Veloski, J. J., & Hojat, M. (1982). Professional attitudes and interpersonal relationships of physicians: Are they a problem? *Proceedings of the Annual Conference on Research in Medical Education, 21*, 117–120. [145].

Herman, M. W., Veloski, J. J., & Hojat, M. (1983). Validity and importance of low ratings given medical graduates in noncognitive areas. *Journal of Medical Education, 58*, 837–843. https://doi.org/10.1097/00001888-198311000-00001 [87].

Hojat, M. (1996). Perception of maternal availability in childhood and selected psychosocial characteristics in adulthood. *Genetic, Social, and General Psychology Monographs, 122*, 425–450. https://pubmed.ncbi.nlm.nih.gov/8976598/ [146].

Hojat, M. (1998). Satisfaction with early relationships with parents and psychosocial attributes in adulthood; Which parent contributes more? *Journal of Genetic Psychology, 159*, 203–220. https://doi.org/10.1080/00221329809596146 [147].

Hojat, M. (2012). Viewpoint: Guiding medical students toward empathetic patient care. *AAMC Reporter, 21*(6), 3. (Published Interview). [228].

Hojat, M. (2014). Assessments of empathy in medical school admissions: What additional evidence is needed? *International Journal of Medical Education, 5*, 7–10. https://doi.org/10.5116/ijme.52b7.5294 [18].

Hojat, M. (2018). Change in empathy in medical school (Letter to the Editor). *Medical Education, 52*, 456–457. https://doi.org/10.1111/medu.13497 [184].

Hojat, M., Axelrod, D., Spandorfer, J., & Mangione, S. (2013a). Enhancing and sustaining empathy in medical students. *Medical Teacher, 35*(12), 996–1001. https://doi.org/10.3109/0142159X.2013.802300 [185].

Hojat, M., Blacklow, R. S., Robeson, M. R., Veloski, J. J., & Borenstein, B. D. (1990a). Postbaccalaureate preparation and performance in medical school. *Academic Medicine, 65*, 388–391. https://journals.lww.com/academicmedicine/Abstract/1990/06000/Postbaccalaureate_preparation_and_performance_in.7.aspx [19].

Hojat, M., Borenstein, B. D., & Veloski, J. J. (1988a). Cognitive and noncognitive factors in predicting the clinical performance of medical school graduates. *Journal of Medical Education, 63*, 323–325. https://doi.org/10.1097/00001888-198804000-00009 [88].

Hojat, M., Brigham, T. P., Gottheil, E., Xu, G., Glaser, K., & Veloski, J. J. (1998). Medical students' personal values and their career choices a quarter-century later. *Psychological Reports, 83*, 243–248. https://doi.org/10.2466/pr0.1998.83.1.243 [148].

Hojat, M., Callahan, C. A., & Gonnella, J. S. (2004a). Students' personality and ratings of clinical competence in medical school clerkships: A longitudinal study. *Psychology, Health & Medicine, 9*, 247–252. https://doi.org/10.1080/13548500410001670771 [149].

Hojat, M., DeSantis, J., & Gonnella, J. S. (2017). Patient perceptions of clinician's empathy: Measurement and psychometrics. *Journal of Patient Experience, 4*(2), 78–83. https://doi.org/10.1177/2374373517699273 [186].

Hojat, M., DeSantis, J., Ney, D. B., & DeCleene-Do, H. (2020). Empathy of medical students and compassionate care for dying patients: An assessment of "No One Dies Alone" program. *Journal of Patient Experience, 7*(6), 1164–1168. https://doi.org/10.1177/2374373520962605 [187].

Hojat, M., Erdmann, J. B., & Gonnella, J. S. (2014). *AMEE Guide 79: Personality assessments and outcomes in medical education and the practice of medicine*. Association for Medical Education in Europe (AMEE). Reprinted as an independent book from the following invited article: Hojat M., Erdmann, J. B., Gonnella. J. S. (2014). Personality assessments and outcomes in medical education and the practice of medicine: AMEE Guide No. 79. *Medical Teacher, 35*(7), e1267–e1301. https://doi.org/10.3109/0142159X.2013.785654 [150].

Hojat, M., Erdmann, J. B., Veloski, J. J., Nasca, T. J., Callahan, C. A., Julian, E., & Peck, J. (2000a). A validity study of the writing sample section of the Medical College Admission

Test. *Academic Medicine, 75*(Supplement), 25–27. https://journals.lww.com/academicmedi-cine/Fulltext/2000/10001/A_Validity_Study_of_the_Writing_Sample_Section_of.8.aspx [6].

Hojat, M., Fields, S. K., & Gonnella, J. S. (2003a). Empathy: An NP/MD comparison. *The Nurse Practitioner, 28*, 45–47. https://doi.org/10.1097/00006205-200304000-00010 [188].

Hojat, M., Fields, S. K., Rattner, S. L., Griffiths, M., Cohen, M. J. M., & Plumb, J. D. (1997). Attitudes toward physician-nurse alliance: Comparisons of medical and nursing students. *Academic Medicine, 72*(Supplement), 1–3. https://doi.org/10.1097/00001888-199710001-00001 [189].

Hojat, M., Fields, S. K., Veloski, J. J., Griffiths, M., Cohen, M. J. M., & Plumb, J. D. (1999a). Psychometric properties of an attitude scale measuring physician-nurse collaboration. *Evaluation & the Health Professions, 22*, 208–220. https://journals.sagepub.com/doi/10.1177/01632789922034275 [190].

Hojat, M., Glaser, K., Xu, G., Veloski, J. J., & Christian, E. B. (1999b). Gender comparisons of medical students' psychosocial profiles. *Medical Education, 33*, 342–349. http://www.blackwell-synergy.com/doi/abs/10.1046/j.1365-2923.1999.00331.x [35].

Hojat, M., Glaser, K. M., & Veloski, J. J. (1996a). Associations between selected psychosocial attributes and ratings of physician competence. *Academic Medicine, 71*(Supplement), S103–S105. https://doi.org/10.1097/00001888-199610000-00059 [151].

Hojat, M., & Gonnella, J. S. (2011). An instrument for measuring pharmacist and physician attitudes towards collaboration: Preliminary psychometric data. *Journal of Interprofessional Care, 25*(1), 66–72. https://doi.org/10.3109/13561820.2010.483368 [191].

Hojat, M., & Gonnella, J. S. (2015). Eleven years of data on the Jefferson Scale of Empathy-Medical student version (JSE-S): Proxy norm data and tentative cutoff scores. *Medical Principles and Practice, 24*, 344–350. https://doi.org/10.1159/000381954 [192].

Hojat, M., & Gonnella, J. S. (2017a). In reply to Quinn and Zelenski (Letter to the Editor). *Academic Medicine, 92*(9), 1219. https://doi.org/10.1097/ACM.0000000000001853 [193].

Hojat, M., & Gonnella, J. S. (2017b). What matters more about the Interpersonal Reactivity Index and the Jefferson Scale of Empathy? Their underlying constructs or their relationships with pertinent measures of clinical competence and patient outcomes? (Invited Commentary). *Academic Medicine, 92*(6), 743–745. https://doi.org/10.1097/ACM.0000000000001424 [194].

Hojat, M., Gonnella, J. S., Erdmann, J. B., Rattner, S. L., Veloski, J. J., Glaser, K., & Xu, G. (2000b). Gender comparisons of income expectations in the USA at the beginning of medical school during the past twenty-eight years. *Social Science & Medicine, 50*, 1665–1672. https://doi.org/10.1016/S0277-9536(99)00407-4 [36].

Hojat, M., Gonnella, J. S., Erdmann, J. B., & Veloski, J. J. (1996b). The fate of medical students with different levels of knowledge: Are the basic medical sciences relevant to physician competence? *Advances in Health Sciences Education, 1*, 179–196. https://link.springer.com/article/10.1007/BF00162915 [51].

Hojat, M., Gonnella, J. S., Erdmann, J. B., Veloski, J. J., Louis, D. Z., Nasca, T. J., & Rattner, S. L. (2000c). Physicians' perceptions of the changing healthcare system: Comparisons by gender and specialties. *Journal of Community Health, 25*, 455–471. https://doi.org/10.1023/a:1005192613992 [152].

Hojat, M., Gonnella, J. S., Erdmann, J. B., Veloski, J. J., & Xu, G. (1995a). Primary care and non-primary care physicians: A longitudinal study of their similarities, differences, and correlates before, during, and after medical school. *Academic Medicine, 70*(Supplement), S17–S28. https://doi.org/10.1097/00001888-199501000-00020 [103].

Hojat, M., Gonnella, J. S., Erdmann, J. B., & Vogel, W. H. (2003b). Medical student's cognitive appraisal of stressful life events as related to personality, physical well-being, and academic performance: A longitudinal study. *Personality and Individual Differences, 35*, 219–235. https://doi.org/10.1016/S0191-8869(02)00186-1 [153].

Hojat, M., Gonnella, J. S., Mangione, S., Nasca, T. J., & Magee, M. (2003c). Physician empathy in medical education and practice: Experience with the Jefferson Scale of Physician Empathy. *Seminars in Integrative Medicine, 1*, 25–41. https://doi.org/10.1016/S1543-1150(03)00002-4 [195].

Hojat, M., Gonnella, J. S., Mangione, S., Nasca, T. J., Veloski, J. J., Erdmann, J. B., Callahan, C. A., & Magee, M. (2002). Empathy in medical students as related to academic performance, clinical competence, and gender. *Medical Education, 36*, 522–527. https://doi.org/10.1046/j.1365-2923.2002.01234.x [196].

Hojat, M., Gonnella, J. S., Nasca, T. J., Fields, S. K., Cicchetti, A., Lo Scalzo, A., Taroni, F., Amicosante, A. M. V., Macinati, M., Tangucci, M., Liva, C., Ricciardi, G., Eidelman, S., Admi, H., Geva, H., Mashiach, T., Alroy, G., Alcorta-Gonzalez, A., Ibarra, D., & Torres-Ruiz, A. (2003d). Comparisons of American, Israeli, Italian and Mexican physicians and nurses on the total and factor scores of the Jefferson Scale of attitudes toward physician-nurse collaborative relationships. *International Journal of Nursing Studies, 40*, 427–435. https://doi.org/10.1016/S0020-7489(02)00108-6 [197].

Hojat, M., Gonnella, J. S., Nasca, T. J., Mangione, S., Veloski, J. J., & Magee, M. (2002a). The Jefferson Scale of Physician Empathy: Further psychometric data and differences by gender and specialty at item level. *Academic Medicine, 77*(Supplement), 58–60. https://doi.org/10.1097/00001888-200210001-00019 [198].

Hojat, M., Gonnella, J. S., Nasca, T. J., Mangione, S., Vergare, M., & Magee, M. (2002b). Physician empathy: Definition, components, measurement, and relationship to gender and specialty. *American Journal of Psychiatry, 159*, 1563–1569. https://doi.org/10.1176/appi.ajp.159.9.1563 [199].

Hojat, M., Gonnella, J. S., & Veloski, J. J. (2010a). Rebuttals to critics of studies of the decline of empathy. *Academic Medicine, 85*(12), 1812; author reply 1813–1814. https://doi.org/10.1097/acm.0b013e3181fa3576 [200].

Hojat, M., Gonnella, J. S., Veloski, J. J., & Erdmann, J. B. (1993a). Is the glass half full or half empty? A reexamination of the associations between assessment measures during medical school and clinical competence after graduation. *Academic Medicine, 68*(Supplement), S69–S76. https://doi.org/10.1097/00001888-199302000-00035 [89].

Hojat, M., Gonnella, J. S., Veloski, J. J., & Erdmann, J. B. (1996c). Jefferson Medical College Longitudinal Study: A prototype for evaluation of changes. *Education for Health, 9*, 99–113. [229].

Hojat, M., Gonnella, J. S., Veloski, J. J., & Moses, S. (1990b). Differences in professional activities, perceptions of professional problems, and practice patterns between men and women graduates of Jefferson Medical College. *Academic Medicine, 65*, 755–761. https://doi.org/10.1097/00001888-199012000-00011 [104].

Hojat, M., Gonnella, J. S., Veloski, J. J., & Xu, G. (1995b). Salary inequities and health-care costs (Letter to the Editor). *Academic Medicine, 70*, 853–854. https://doi.org/10.1097/00001888-199510000-00001 [37].

Hojat, M., Gonnella, J. S., & Xu, G. (1995c). Gender comparisons of young physicians' perceptions of their medical education, professional life, and practice: A follow-up study of Jefferson Medical College graduates. *Academic Medicine, 70*, 305–312. https://doi.org/10.1097/00001888-199504000-00014 [38].

Hojat, M., & Herman, M. W. (1985). Developing an instrument to measure attitudes toward nurses: Preliminary psychometric findings. *Psychological Reports, 56*, 571–579. https://doi.org/10.2466/pr0.1985.56.2.571 [201].

Hojat, M., Kowitt, B., Doria, C., & Gonnella, J. S. (2010b). Career satisfaction and professional accomplishments. *Medical Education, 44*(10), 969–976. https://doi.org/10.1111/j.1365-2923.2010.03735.x [154].

Hojat, M., & LaNoue, M. (2014). Exploration and confirmation of the latent variable structure of the Jefferson Scale of Empathy. *International Journal of Medical Education, 5*, 73–81. https://doi.org/10.5116/ijme.533f.0c41 [202].

Hojat, M., Louis, D., Maxwell, K., & Gonnella, J. (2011a). The Jefferson Scale of Empathy (JSE): An update. *Population Health Matters (Formerly Health Policy Newsletter), 24*(2), 5–6. https://jdc.jefferson.edu/cgi/viewcontent.cgi?article=1727&context=hpn [203].

Hojat, M., Louis, D. Z., Maio, V., & Gonnella, J. S. (2013b). Editorial: Empathy and health care quality. *American Journal of Medical Quality, 28*(1), 6–7. https://doi.org/10.1177/1062860612464731 [204].

Hojat, M., & Lyons, K. (1998). Psychosocial characteristics of female students in the allied health and medical colleges: Psychometrics of the measures and personality profiles. *Advances in Health Sciences Education, 3*, 119–132. https://doi.org/10.1023/A:1009733623166 [155].

Hojat, M., Mangione, S., Gonnella, J. S., Nasca, T. J., Veloski, J. J., & Kane, G. (2001a). Empathy in medical education and patient care (Letter to the Editor). *Academic Medicine, 76*, 669. https://journals.lww.com/academicmedicine/Fulltext/2001/07000/Empathy_in_Medical_Education_and_Patient_Care.1.aspx [205].

Hojat, M., Mangione, S., Kane, G. C., & Gonnella, J. S. (2005a). Relationships between scores of the Jefferson Scale of Physician Empathy (JSPE) and the Interpersonal Reactivity Index (IRI). *Medical Teacher, 27*, 625–628. https://doi.org/10.1080/01421590500069744 [206].

Hojat, M., Mangione, S., Nasca, T. J., Cohen, M. J. M., Gonnella, J. S., Erdmann, J. B., Veloski, J. J., & Magee, M. (2001b). The Jefferson Scale of Physician Empathy: Development and preliminary psychometric data. *Educational and Psychological Measurement, 61*, 349–365. http://epm.sagepub.com/cgi/content/abstract/61/2/349 [207].

Hojat, M., Mangione, S., Nasca, T. J., Gonnella, J. S., & Magee, M. (2005b). Empathy scores in medical school and ratings of empathic behavior in residency training 3 years later. *The Journal of Social Psychology, 145*(6), 663–672. https://doi.org/10.3200/SOCP.145.6.663-672 [156].

Hojat, M., Mangione, S., Nasca, T. J., Rattner, S. L., Erdmann, J. B., Gonnella, J. S., & Magee, M. (2004b). An empirical study of decline in empathy in medical school. *Medical Education, 38*, 934–941. https://doi.org/10.1111/j.1365-2929.2004.01911.x [208].

Hojat, M., Michalec, B., Veloski, J. J., & Tykocinski, M. L. (2015a). Can empathy, other personality attributes, and level of positive social influence in medical school identify potential leaders in medicine? *Academic Medicine, 90*, 505–510. https://doi.org/10.1097/ACM.0000000000000652 [157].

Hojat, M., Nasca, T. J., Cohen, M. J. M., Fields, S. K., Rattner, S. L., Griffiths, M., Ibarra, D., de Gonzalez, A. A., Torres-Ruiz, A., Ibarra, G., & Garcia, A. (2001c). Attitudes toward physician-nurse collaboration: A cross-cultural study of male and female physicians and nurses in the United States and Mexico. *Nursing Research, 50*, 123–128. https://doi.org/10.1097/00006199-200103000-00008 [209].

Hojat, M., Nasca, T. J., Erdmann, J. B., Frisby, A. J., Veloski, J. J., & Gonnella, J. S. (2003e). An operational measure of physician lifelong learning: Its development, components and preliminary psychometric data. *Medical Teacher, 25*, 433–437. https://doi.org/10.1080/0142159031000137463 [210].

Hojat, M., Nasca, T. J., Magee, M., Feeney, K., Pascual, R., Urbano, F., & Gonnella, J. S. (1999c). A comparison of the personality profiles of internal medicine residents, physician role models, and the general population. *Academic Medicine, 74*, 54–60. https://doi.org/10.1097/00001888-199912000-00017 [158].

Hojat, M., Paskin, D. L., Callahan, C. A., Nasca, T. J., Louis, D. Z., Veloski, J., Erdmann, J. B., & Gonnella, J. S. (2007). Components of postgraduate competence: Analyses of thirty years of longitudinal data. *Medical Education, 41*(10), 982–989. https://doi.org/10.1111/j.1365-2923.2007.02841 [90].

Hojat, M., Robeson, M. R., Damjanov, I., Veloski, J. J., Glaser, K., & Gonnella, J. S. (1993b). Students' psychosocial characteristics as predictors of academic performance in medical school. *Academic Medicine, 68*, 635–637. https://doi.org/10.1097/00001888-199308000-00015 [159].

Hojat, M., Robeson, M. R., Veloski, J. J., Blacklow, R. S., Xu, G., & Gonnella, J. S. (1994). Gender comparisons prior to, during, and after medical school using two decades of longitudinal data at Jefferson Medical College. *Evaluation & the Health Professions, 17*, 290–306. https://doi.org/10.1177/016327879401700303 [39].

Hojat, M., Spandorfer, J., Isenberg, G. A., Vergare, M. J., Fassihi, R., & Gonnella, J. S. (2012). Psychometrics of the scale of attitudes toward physician-pharmacist collaboration: A study with medical students. *Medical Teacher, 34*(12), e833–e837. https://doi.org/10.3109/0142159X.2012.714877 [211].

Hojat, M., Spandorfer, J., Louis, D. Z., & Gonnella, J. S. (2011b). Empathic and sympathetic orientations toward patient care: Conceptualization, measurement, and psychometrics. *Academic Medicine, 86*(8), 989–995. https://doi.org/10.1097/ACM.0b013e31822203d8 [160].

Hojat, M., Veloski, J., Nasca, T. J., Erdmann, J. B., & Gonnella, J. S. (2006). Assessing physicians' orientation toward lifelong learning. *Journal of General Internal Medicine, 21*(9), 931–936. https://doi.org/10.1111/j.1525-1497.2006.00500.x [214].

Hojat, M., & Veloski, J. J. (1984). Subtest scores of a comprehensive examination of medical knowledge as a function of retention interval. *Psychological Reports, 55,* 579–585. https://doi.org/10.2466/pr0.1984.55.2.579 [58].

Hojat, M., Veloski, J. J., & Borenstein, B. D. (1986). Components of clinical competence ratings of physicians: An empirical approach. *Educational and Psychological Measurement, 46,* 761–769. https://doi.org/10.1177/0013164486463034 [91].

Hojat, M., Veloski, J. J., & Gonnella, J. S. (2009a). Measurement and correlates of physicians' lifelong learning. *Academic Medicine, 84*(8), 1066–1074. https://doi.org/10.1097/ACM.0b013e3181acf25f [212].

Hojat, M., Veloski, J. J., & Gonnella, J. S. (2010c). Physician lifelong learning: Conceptualization, measurement, and correlates in full-time clinicians and academic clinicians. In M. P. Caltone (Ed.), *Handbook of lifelong learning development* (pp. 37–78). Nova Science Publishers. This book chapter was reprinted with minor modifications in: Hojat, M., Veloski, J. J., & Gonnella, J. S. (2012). Physician lifelong learning: Conceptualization, measurement, and correlates in full-time clinicians, academic clinicians, and medical students. In Neimeyer, G. J., & Taylor, J. M. (Eds.) *Continuing professional development and lifelong learning issues, impacts and outcomes* (pp. 29–70). Nova Science Publishers. https://www.researchgate.net/publication/326244935_Physician_lifelong_learning_Conceptualization_measurement_and_correlates_in_full-time_clinicians_and_academic_clinicians [213].

Hojat, M., Veloski, J. J., Gonnella, J. S., Erdmann, J. B., & Rattner, S. L. (1999d). Attitudes toward managed care: A brief instrument to measure attitudes of medical students towards change in the healthcare system. *Academic Medicine, 74*(Supplement), 78–80. https://doi.org/10.1097/00001888-199910000-00046 [161].

Hojat, M., Veloski, J. J., Louis, D. Z., Xu, G., Ibarra, D., Gottlieb, J. E., & Erdmann, J. B. (1999e). Perceptions of medical school seniors of the current changes in the U.S. healthcare system. *Evaluation & the Health Professions, 22,* 169–183. https://journals.sagepub.com/doi/10.1177/01632789922034248 [162].

Hojat, M., Veloski, J. J., & Zeleznik, C. (1985). Predictive validity of the MCAT for students with two sets of scores. *Journal of Medical Education, 60,* 911–918. https://doi.org/10.1097/00001888-198512000-00002 [7].

Hojat, M., Vergare, M., Isenberg, G., Cohen, M., & Spandorfer, J. (2015b). Underlying construct of empathy, optimism, and burnout in medical students. *International Journal of Medical Education, 6,* 12–16. https://doi.org/10.5116/ijme.54c3.60cd [163].

Hojat, M., Vergare, M. J., Maxwell, K., Brainard, G., Herrine, S. K., Isenberg, G. A., Veloski, J., & Gonnella, J. S. (2009b). The devil is in the third year: A longitudinal study of erosion of empathy in medical school. *Academic Medicine, 84*(9), 1182–1191. https://doi.org/10.1097/ACM.0b013e3181b17e55 [164].

Hojat, M., Vogel, W. H., Zeleznik, C., & Borenstein, B. D. (1988b). Effects of academic and psychosocial predictors of performance in medical school on coefficients of determination. *Psychological Reports, 63,* 383–394. https://doi.org/10.2466/pr0.1988.63.2.383 [165].

Hojat, M., Ward, J., Spandorfer, J., Arenson, C., Van Winkle, L. J., & Williams, B. (2015c). The Jefferson Scale of Attitudes Toward Interprofessional Collaboration (JeffSATIC): Development and multi-institution psychometric data. *Journal of Interprofessional Care, 29,* 238–244. https://doi.org/10.3109/13561820.2014.962129 [215].

Hojat, M., & Zuckerman, M. (2008). Personality and specialty interest in medical students. *Medical Teacher, 30,* 400–406. https://doi.org/10.1080/01421590802043835 [166].

Hojat, M., Zuckerman, M., Gonnella, J. S., Mangione, S., Nasca, T. J., Vergare, M., & Magee, M. (2005c). Empathy in medical students as related to specialty interest, personality, and perceptions of mother and father. *Personality and Individual Differences, 39*, 1205–1215. https://doi.org/10.1016/j.paid.2005.04.007 [216].

Isenberg, G., Brown, A. M., DeSantis, J., Veloski, J., & Hojat, M. (2020). The relationship between grit and selected personality measures in medical students. *International Journal of Medical Education, 11*, 25–30. https://doi.org/10.5116/ijme.5e01.f32d [167].

Isenberg, G. A., Roy, V., Veloski, J., Berg, K., & Yeo, C. J. (2015). Evaluation of the validity of medical students' self-assessments of proficiency in clinical simulations. *The Journal of Surgical Research, 193*(2), 554–559. https://doi.org/10.1016/j.jss.2014.09.036 [59].

Kusurkar, R. A., & Croiset, G. (2016). Creating a longitudinal database in medical education: Perspectives from the pioneers. *Education for Health, 29*, 266–270. https://doi.org/10.4103/1357-6283.204214 (Published Interview). [230].

Lo Sasso, A. A., Lamberton, C. E., Sammon, M., Berg, K. T., Caruso, J. W., Cass, J., & Hojat, M. (2017). Enhancing student empathetic engagement, history-taking, and communication skills during electronic medical record use in patient care. *Academic Medicine, 92*(7), 1022–1027. https://doi.org/10.1097/ACM.0000000000001476 [217].

Louis, D. Z., Gottlieb, J., Markham, F. W., Hojat, M., Rabinowitz, C., & Gonnella, J. S. (1996). Students' gender and examination of patients in a third-year family medicine clerkship. *Academic Medicine, 71*(Supplement), S19–S21. https://doi.org/10.1097/00001888-199610000-00032 [60].

Mangione, S., Kane, G. C., Caruso, J. W., Gonnella, J. S., Nasca, T. J., & Hojat, M. (2002). Assessment of empathy in different years of internal medicine training. *Medical Teacher, 24*, 370–373. https://doi.org/10.1080/01421590220145725 [218].

Markham, F. W., Rattner, S. L., Hojat, M., Louis, D. Z., Rabinowitz, C., & Gonnella, J. S. (2002). Evaluations of medical students' clinical experiences in a family medicine clerkship: Differences in patient encounters by disease severity in different clerkship sites. *Family Medicine, 34*, 451–454. https://europepmc.org/article/med/12164623 [61].

Michalec, B., Veloski, J. J., & Hafferty, F. (2016). Predicting peer nominations among medical students: A social network approach. *Academic Medicine, 91*(6), 847–852. https://doi.org/10.1097/ACM.0000000000001079 [168].

Michalec, B., Veloski, J. J., Hojat, M., & Tykocinski, M. L. (2015). Identifying potential engaging leaders within medical education: The role of positive influence on peers. *Medical Teacher, 37*(7), 677–683. https://doi.org/10.3109/0142159X.2014.947933 [169].

Modi, A., Fascelli, M., Daitch, Z., & Hojat, M. (2017). Evaluating the relationship between participation in student-run free clinics and changes in empathy in medical students. *Journal of Primary Care & Community Health, 8*(3), 122–126. https://doi.org/10.1177/2150131916685199 [219].

Nasca, T. J., Gonnella, J. S., Hojat, M., Veloski, J. J., Erdmann, J. B., Robeson, M. R., Brigham, T. P., & Callahan, C. A. (2002). Conceptualization and measurement of clinical competence of residents: A brief rating form and its psychometric properties. *Medical Teacher, 24*, 299–303. https://doi.org/10.1080/01421590220134141 [92].

Nicholson, S. (2005). How much do medical students know about physician income? *The Journal of Human Resources, 40*, 100–114. http://jhr.uwpress.org/content/XL/1/100.short [170].

Novielli, K., Hojat, M., Park, P. K., Gonnella, J. S., & Veloski, J. J. (2001). Change of interest in surgery during medical school: A comparison of men and women. *Academic Medicine, 76*(Supplement), 58–61. https://doi.org/10.1097/00001888-200110001-00020 [40].

Novielli, K. D., Hojat, M., Nasca, T. J., Erdmann, J. B., & Veloski, J. J. (2000). Correlates of physicians' endorsement of the legalization of physician-assisted suicide. *Academic Medicine, 75*(Supplement), 53–55. https://doi.org/10.1097/00001888-200010001-00017 [171].

Papadakis, M. A., Teherani, A., Banach, M. A., Knettler, T. R., Rattner, S. L., Stern, D. T., Veloski, J. J., & Hodgson, C. S. (2005). Disciplinary action by medical boards and prior behavior in medical school. *The New England Journal of Medicine, 353*(25), 2673–2682. https://doi.org/10.1056/NEJMsa052596 [231].

Pohl, C. A., Hojat, M., & Arnold, L. (2011). Peer nominations as related to academic attainment, empathy, personality, and specialty interest. *Academic Medicine, 86*(6), 747–751. https://doi. org/10.1097/ACM.0b013e318217e464 [172].

Pohl, C. A., Robeson, M. R., Hojat, M., Rattner, S. L., & Veloski, J. J. (2002). Sooner or later? USMLE Step 1 performance and test administration date at the end of the second year. *Academic Medicine, 77*(Supplement), S17–S19. http://www.academicmedicine.org/pt/re/ acmed/pdfhandler.00001888-200210001-00006.pdf [52].

Pohl, C. A., Robeson, M. R., & Veloski, J. J. (2004). USMLE Step 2 performance and test administration date in the fourth year of medical school. *Academic Medicine, 79*(Supplement), S49–S51. https://doi.org/10.1097/00001888-200410001-00015 [62].

Rabinowitz, H. K. (1983). A program to recruit and educate medical students to practice family medicine in underserved areas. *Journal of the American Medical Association, 249*, 1038–1041. https://jamanetwork.com/journals/jama/fullarticle/383947 [20].

Rabinowitz, H. K. (1988). Evaluation of a selective medical school admissions policy to increase the number of family physicians in rural and underserved areas. *The New England Journal of Medicine, 319*, 480–486. https://www.nejm.org/doi/full/10.1056/ NEJM198808253190805 [21].

Rabinowitz, H. K., Diamond, J. J., Hojat, M., & Hazelwood, C. E. (1999a). Demographic, educational, and economic factors related to recruitment and retention of physicians in rural Pennsylvania. *The Journal of Rural Health, 15*, 212–218. https://doi.org/10.1111/j.1748-0361.1999.tb00742.x [22].

Rabinowitz, H. K., Diamond, J. J., Markham, F. W., & Hazelwood, C. E. (1999b). A program to increase the number of family physicians in rural and underserved areas: Impact after 22 years. *Journal of the American Medical Association, 281*, 255–260. https://doi.org/10.1001/ jama.281.3.255 [105].

Rabinowitz, H. K., Diamond, J. J., Markham, F. W., & Paynter, N. P. (2001). Critical factors for designing programs to increase the supply and retention of rural primary care physicians. *Journal of the American Medical Association, 286*, 1041–1048. https://doi.org/10.1001/ jama.286.9.1041 [106].

Rabinowitz, H. K., & Hojat, M. (1989). A comparison of the modified essay question and multiple choice question formats: Their relationships to clinical performance. *Family Medicine, 21*, 364–367. https://pubmed.ncbi.nlm.nih.gov/2792608/ [63].

Rabinowitz, H. K., Hojat, M., Veloski, J. J., Rattner, S. L., Robeson, M. R., Xu, G., Appel, M. H., Cochran, C., Jones, R. L., & Kanter, S. L. (1999c). Who is a generalist? An analysis of whether physicians trained as generalists practice as generalists. *Evaluation & the Health Profession, 22*, 539–544. https://doi.org/10.1177/016327879902200406 [107].

Rabinowitz, H. K., Veloski, J. J., Aber, R. C., Adler, S., Ferretti, S., Kelliher, G. J., Mochen, E., Morrison, G., Rattner, S. L., Sterling, G., Robeson, M. R., Hojat, M., & Xu, G. (1999d). A statewide system to track medical students' careers: The Pennsylvania model. *Academic Medicine, 74*(Supplement), S112–S118. https://doi.org/10.1097/00001888-199901001-00042 [108].

Rabinowitz, H. K., Xu, G., Robeson, M. R., Hojat, M., Rattner, S. L., Appel, M. H., Cochran, C., Johnson, J. J., Kanter, S. L., & Veloski, J. J. (1997). Generalist career plans: Tracking medical school seniors through residency. *Academic Medicine, 72*, 103–105. https://doi. org/10.1097/00001888-199710001-00035 [109].

Rabinowitz, H. K., Xu, G., Veloski, J. J., Rattner, S. L., Robeson, M. R., Hojat, M., Appel, M. H., Cochran, C., Jones, R. L., & Kanter, S. L. (2000). Choice of first-year residency position and long-term generalist career choices (Letter to the Editor). *Journal of the American Medical Association, 284*, 1081–1082. https://pubmed.ncbi.nlm.nih.gov/10974685/ [110].

Rattner, S. L., Louis, D. Z., Rabinowitz, C., Gottlieb, J. E., Nasca, T. J., Markham, F. W., Gottlieb, R. P., Caruso, J. W., Lane, J. L., Veloski, J., Hojat, M., & Gonnella, J. S. (2001). Documenting and comparing medical students' clinical experiences. *Journal of the American Medical Association, 286*, 1035–1040. http://jama.ama-assn.org/cgi/content/ abstract/286/9/1035 [64].

Rattner, S. L., Robeson, M. R., & Veloski, J. J. (1997). Assessment of physicians' interest in primary care training/retraining. *Academic Medicine, 72*, 1103–1105. https://doi.org/10.1097/00001888-199712000-00023 [111].

Rimoldi, H. A., Raimondo, R., Erdmann, J. B., & Hojat, M. (2002). Intra- and intercultural comparisons of personality profiles of medical students in Argentina and the United States. *Adolescence, 37*, 477–494. https://pubmed.ncbi.nlm.nih.gov/12458688/ [173].

Rodgers, J. F., Veloski, J. J., & Moses, S. (1987). Student ratings of clerkship activities as a basis for curriculum modification: A four year comparison of six departments. *Proceedings of the Twenty-Sixth Annual Conference on Research in Medical Education, 26*, 179–184. https://europepmc.org/article/med/3454583 [65].

Rosenfeld, L. M., Hojat, M., Veloski, J. J., Blacklow, R. S., & Goepp, C. E. (1992). Delays in completing medical school: Predictors and outcomes. *Teaching and Learning in Medicine, 4*, 162–167. https://www.tandfonline.com/doi/abs/10.1080/10401339209539556 [8].

Rosenthal, M. P., Turner, T. N., Diamond, J. J., & Rabinowitz, H. K. (1992). Income expectations of first-year students at Jefferson Medical College as a predictor of family practice specialty choice. *Academic Medicine, 67*, 328–331. https://doi.org/10.1097/00001888-199205000-00012 [175].

Rosenthal, S., Schlussel, Y., Yaden, M. B., DeSantis, J., Trayes, K., Pohl, C., & Hojat, M. (2021). Persistent impostor phenomenon is associated with distress in medical students. *Family Medicine, 53*(2), 118–122. https://doi.org/10.22454/FamMed.2021.799997 [174].

Rosenthal, S. R., Russo, S., Berg, K., Majdan, J., Wilson, J., Grinberg, C., & Veloski, J. J. (2019). Identifying students at risk of failing the USMLE Step 2 Clinical Skills Examination. *Family Medicine, 51*(6), 483–499. https://doi.org/10.22454/FamMed.2019.429968 [66].

Rosenzweig, S., Reibel, D. K., Greeson, J. M., Brainair, G. C., & Hojat, M. (2003). Mindfulness-based stress reduction lowers psychological distress in medical students. *Teaching and Learning in Medicine, 15*, 88–92. https://doi.org/10.1207/S15328015TLM1502_03 [176].

Schwartz, G. F., Veloski, J. J., & Gonnella, J. S. (1976). Evaluation of the surgical clerkship experience in affiliated hospitals: Performance on objective examinations. *Journal of Surgical Research, 20*, 179–182. https://doi.org/10.1016/0022-4804(76)90137-2 [67].

Seltzer, J. L., & Veloski, J. J. (1982). Changing specialties: Do anesthesiologists differ from other physicians? *Anesthesia and Analgesia, 61*, 504–506. https://pubmed.ncbi.nlm.nih.gov/7200739/ [112].

Seltzer, J. L., & Veloski, J. J. (1983). Migration of physicians to and from anesthesiology (Letter to the Editor). *Anesthesia and Analgesia, 62*, 702. https://journals.lww.com/anesthesia-analgesia/Citation/1983/07000/Migration_of_Physicians_to_and_from.18.aspx [113].

Sierles, F. S., Vergare, M. J., Hojat, M., & Gonnella, J. S. (2004). Academic performance of psychiatrists compared to other specialists before, during, and after medical school. *American Journal of Psychiatry, 161*, 1477–1482. https://doi.org/10.1176/appi.ajp.161.8.1477 [114].

Silber, C., & Veloski, J. J. (2005). Board certification in obstetrics and gynecology: Associations with physicians' demographics and performances during medical school. *American Journal of Obstetrics and Gynecology, 192*, 318–322. https://doi.org/10.1016/j.ajog.2004.09.007 [68].

Silber, C. G., Nasca, T. J., Paskin, D. L., Eiger, G., Robeson, M. R., & Veloski, J. J. (2004). Do global rating forms enable program directors to assess the ACGME Competencies? *Academic Medicine, 79*, 549–556. https://doi.org/10.1097/00001888-200406000-00010 [115].

Swanson, D. B., Case, S. M., Waechter, D., Veloski, J. J., Hasbrouck, C., Friedman, M., Carline, J. D., & Maclaren, C. (1993). A preliminary study of the validity of scores and pass/fail standards for USMLE Steps 1 and 2. *Academic Medicine, 68*(Supplement), S19–S21. https://doi.org/10.1097/00001888-199310000-00033 [69].

Turner, B. J., Hojat, M., & Gonnella, J. S. (1987). Using ratings of resident competence to evaluate NBME examination passing standards. *Journal of Medical Education, 62*, 572–581. https://doi.org/10.1097/00001888-198707000-00006 [53].

Veloski, J. J. (1979). Using postgraduate clinical performance to monitor change in the medical school. *Proceedings of the Eighteenth Annual Conference on Research in Medical Education, Washington, DC* (p. 425). [23].

Veloski, J. J., Callahan, C. A., Xu, G., Hojat, M., & Nash, D. B. (2000). Prediction of students' performance on licensing examinations using age, race, sex, undergraduate GPAs and MCAT scores. *Academic Medicine, 75*(Supplement), S28–S30. https://doi. org/10.1097/00001888-200010001-00009 [41].

Veloski, J. J., Fields, S. K., Boex, J. R., & Blank, L. L. (2005). Measuring professionalism: A review of studies with instruments reported in the literature between 1982 and 2002. *Academic Medicine, 80*, 366–370. https://doi.org/10.1097/00001888-200504000-00014 [220].

Veloski, J. J., Herman, M. W., Gonnella, J. S., Zeleznik, C., & Kellow, W. F. (1979). Relationships between performance in medical school and first postgraduate year. *Journal of Medical Education, 54*, 909–916. https://doi.org/10.1097/00001888-197912000-00001 [93].

Veloski, J. J., Hojat, M., Erdmann, J. B., & Gonnella, J. S. (1998). Affirmative action and special consideration admissions to medical school (Letter to the Editor). *Journal of the American Medical Association, 279*, 508–509. https://jamanetwork.com/journals/jama/fullarticle/1152568 [94].

Veloski, J. J., Hojat, M., & Gonnella, J. (2013). The Jefferson Longitudinal Study of Medical Education: Five decades of outcomes assessment. *Population Health Matters (Formerly Health Policy Newsletter), 26*(1), 2–3. https://jdc.jefferson.edu/hpn/vol26/iss1/3 [232].

Veloski, J. J., Hojat, M., & Gonnella, J. S. (1990). A validity study of Part III of the National Board Examination. *Evaluation & the Health Professions, 13*, 227–240. https://doi. org/10.1177/016327879001300206 [95].

Veloski, J. J., Hojat, M., & Zeleznik, C. (1981a). The overall validity of the new MCAT. In *Proceedings of the Twentieth Annual Conference on Research in Medical Education, Washington, DC* (pp. 129–134) https://pubmed.ncbi.nlm.nih.gov/7347515/ [9].

Veloski, J. J., Zeleznik, C., & Hojat, M. (1981b). The income expectations of medical students in the time period 1970 to 1980. *Proceedings of the Twentieth Annual Conference on Research in Medical Education, 20*, 61–66. https://pubmed.ncbi.nlm.nih.gov/7347546/ [177].

Williams, T., Sachs, L., & Veloski, J. J. (1986). Performance on the NBME Part II examination and career choice. *Journal of Medical Education, 61*, 979–981. https://doi. org/10.1097/00001888-198612000-00006 [116].

Wolfson, P. J., Robeson, M. R., & Veloski, J. J. (1991). Medical students who enter general surgery residency programs: A follow-up between 1972 and 1986. *The American Journal of Surgery, 162*, 491–494. https://doi.org/10.1016/0002-9610(91)90270-n [117].

Worzala, K., Rattner, S. L., Boulet, J. R., Majdan, J. F., Berg, D. D., Robeson, M., & Veloski, J. J. (2008). Evaluation of the congruence between students' post-encounter notes and standardized patients' checklists in a clinical skills examination. *Teaching and Learning in Medicine, 20*(1), 31–36. https://doi.org/10.1080/10401330701798253 [70].

Xu, G., Brigham, T. P., Veloski, J. J., & Rodgers, J. F. (1993a). Attendings' and residents' teaching role and students' overall rating of clinical clerkships. *Medical Teacher, 15*, 217–222. https:// doi.org/10.3109/01421599309006716 [71].

Xu, G., Brigham, T. P., Veloski, J. J., & Rodgers, J. F. (1993b). Perceptions of practice problems encountered by family physicians, pediatricians and orthopedic surgeons. *Evaluation & the Health Professions, 16*, 119–129. https://doi.org/10.1177/016327879301600109 [118].

Xu, G., Hojat, M., Brigham, T. P., Robeson, M. R., & Veloski, J. J. (1994a). Primary care and nonprimary care physicians' concerns in practice and perceptions of medical school curriculum. *Evaluation & the Health Professions, 17*, 436–445. https://doi. org/10.1177/016327879401700405 [119].

Xu, G., Hojat, M., Brigham, T. P., & Veloski, J. J. (1999a). Factors associated with changing levels of interest in primary care during medical school. *Academic Medicine, 74*, 1011–1015. https:// doi.org/10.1097/00001888-199909000-00015 [120].

Xu, G., Hojat, M., & Veloski, J. J. (1994b). Emergency medicine career change: Associations with performances in medical school and in the first postgraduate year and with indebtedness. *Academic Emergency Medicine, 1*, 443–447. https://doi.org/10.1111/j.1553-2712.1994. tb02524.x [121].

Xu, G., Hojat, M., Veloski, J. J., & Brose, J. (1996a). A national study of factors influencing primary care choices among underrepresented-minority, white, and Asian-American physicians. *Academic Medicine, 71*(Supplement), S10–S12. https://doi.org/10.1097/00001888-199610000-00029 [42].

Xu, G., Hojat, M., Veloski, J. J., & Gonnella, J. S. (1999b). The changing healthcare system. A research agenda for medical education. *Evaluation and the Health Professions, 22*, 152–168. https://doi.org/10.1177/01632789922034239 [122].

Xu, G., Rattner, S. L., Veloski, J. J., Hojat, M., Fields, S. K., & Barzansky, B. (1995a). A national study of the factors influencing men and women physicians' choices of primary care specialties. *Academic Medicine, 70*, 398–404. https://doi.org/10.1097/00001888-199505000-00016 [123].

Xu, G., & Veloski, J. J. (1991). A comparison of Jefferson Medical College graduates who chose emergency medicine with those who chose other specialties. *Academic Medicine, 66*, 366–368. https://doi.org/10.1097/00001888-199106000-00014 [124].

Xu, G., & Veloski, J. J. (1992). Factors influencing physicians' decisions to remain in emergency medicine. *Academic Medicine, 67*, 413. https://doi.org/10.1097/00001888-199206000-00016 [125].

Xu, G., & Veloski, J. J. (1993a). Comparing the academic performances of geriatricians and other family physicians and internists. *Academic Medicine, 68*, 388. https://doi.org/10.1097/00001888-199305000-00027 [126].

Xu, G., & Veloski, J. J. (1993b). Influence of previous clerkship experiences on students' satisfaction with their current clerkship. *Academic Medicine, 68*, 230. https://journals.lww.com/academicmedicine/Abstract/1993/03000/Influence_of_previous_clerkship_experiences_on.18.aspx [72].

Xu, G., Veloski, J. J., Barzansky, B., Hojat, M., Diamond, J. J., & Silenzio, V. M. B. (1996b). Comparisons among three types of generalist physicians: Personal characteristics, medical school experiences, financial aid, and other factors influencing career choice. *Advances in Health Sciences Education, 1*, 197–207. https://pubmed.ncbi.nlm.nih.gov/24179019/ [127].

Xu, G., Veloski, J. J., & Brigham, T. P. (1995b). A correlation study of students' perception of their active role as related to their clerkship experiences. *Medical Teacher, 17*, 199–203. https://doi.org/10.3109/01421599509008308 [73].

Xu, G., Veloski, J. J., & Hojat, M. (1993c). Changing interest in family medicine and students' academic performance. *Academic Medicine, 68*(Supplement), S52–S54. https://doi.org/10.1097/00001888-199310000-00044 [128].

Xu, G., Veloski, J. J., & Hojat, M. (1995c). Performance on the NBME Part I examination (Letter to the Editor). *Journal of the American Medical Association, 273*, 617–618. https://journals.lww.com/academicmedicine/abstract/1985/06000/performance_on_nbme_part_i_examination_in_relation.2.aspx [43].

Xu, G., Veloski, J. J., & Hojat, M. (1998). Board certification: Associations with physicians' demographics and performances during medical school and residency. *Academic Medicine, 73*, 1283–1289. https://doi.org/10.1097/00001888-199812000-00019 [44].

Xu, G., Veloski, J. J., Hojat, M., & Fields, S. K. (1995d). Physicians' intention to stay in or leave primary care specialties and variables associated with such intention. *Evaluation & the Health Professions, 18*, 92–102. https://doi.org/10.1177/016327879501800107 [129].

Xu, G., Veloski, J. J., Hojat, M., Gonnella, J. S., & Bacharach, B. (1993d). Longitudinal comparison of the academic performances of Asian-American and white medical students. *Academic Medicine, 68*, 82–86. https://pubmed.ncbi.nlm.nih.gov/8447898/ [45].

Xu, G., Veloski, J. J., Hojat, M., Politzer, R. M., Rabinowitz, H. K., & Rattner, S. L. (1997a). Factors influencing physicians' choices to practice in inner-city or rural areas (Letter to the Editor). *Academic Medicine, 72*, 1026. http://ovidsp.ovid.com/ovidweb.cgi?T=JS&PAGE=reference&D=ovftc&NEWS=N&AN=00001888-199712000-00004 [131].

Xu, G., Veloski, J. J., Hojat, M., Politzer, R. M., Rabinowitz, H. K., & Rattner, S. L. (1997b). Factors influencing primary care physicians' choice to practice in medically underserved areas. *Academic Medicine, 72*(Supplement), 109–111. https://doi.org/10.1097/00001888-199710001-00037 [130].

Yaden, M. E., Yaden, D. B., Buffone, A. E. K., Eichstaedt, J. C., Crutchley, P., Smith, L. K., Cass, J. L., Callahan, C. A., Rosenthal, S. R., Ungar, L. H., Schwartz, H. A., & Hojat, M. (2020). Linguistic analysis of empathy in medical school admission essays. *International Journal of Medical Education, 11*, 186–190. https://www.ijme.net/archive/11/linguistic-analysis-of-empathy/ [221].

Zeleznik, C., Hojat, M., Goepp, C., Amadio, P., Kowlessar, O. D., & Borenstein, B. D. (1988). Students' certainty during course test-taking and performance on clerkships and board exams. *Journal of Medical Education, 63*, 881–891. https://doi.org/10.1097/00001888-198812000-00001 [178].

Zeleznik, C., Hojat, M., & Veloski, J. J. (1983a). Baccalaureate preparation for medical school: Does type of degree make a difference? *Journal of Medical Education, 58*, 26–33. https://pubmed.ncbi.nlm.nih.gov/6848754/#:~:text=No%20significant%20difference%20was%20found,more%20frequently%20than%20the%20others [24].

Zeleznik, C., Hojat, M., & Veloski, J. J. (1983b). Levels of recommendation for students and academic performance in medical school. *Psychological Reports, 52*, 851–858. https://doi.org/10.2466/pr0.1983.52.3.851 [25].

Zeleznik, C., Hojat, M., & Veloski, J. J. (1983c). Long-range predictive and differential validities of the Scholastic Aptitude Test in medical school. *Educational and Psychological Measurement, 43*, 223–232. https://journals.sagepub.com/doi/abs/10.1177/001316448304300129 [10].

Zeleznik, C., Hojat, M., & Veloski, J. J. (1987). Predictive validity of the MCAT as a function of undergraduate institution. *Journal of Medical Education, 62*, 163–169. https://doi.org/10.1097/00001888-198703000-00003 [11].

Zeleznik, C., Veloski, J. J., Conly, S., & Hojat, M. (1980). The relationship between MCAT science subtest scores and performance in medical school: The impact of the undergraduate institution. In *Proceedings of the Nineteenth Annual Conference on Research in Medical Education, Washington, DC* (pp. 257–262) https://pubmed.ncbi.nlm.nih.gov/7458210/ [12].

Name Index

A
Aber, R.C., 108
Adler, S., 108
Admi, H., 197
Alcorta-Gonzalez, A., 197, 209
Alroy, G., 197
Amadio, P., 178
Amicosante, A.M.V., 197
Ankam, N.S., 137
Appel, M.H., 107, 109
Apple, M.H., 110
Arenson, C., 215
Arnold, L., 172
Ashikawa, H., 13, 54
Axelrod, D., 185

B
Bacharach, B., 45
Banach, M.A., 231
Barzansky, B., 123, 127
Bashook, P.G., 85
Berg, D., 30, 55, 56, 182
Berg, D.D., 70
Berg, K., 30, 55, 56, 59, 66, 182
Berg, K.T., 217
Blacklow, R.S., 5, 8, 19, 39, 79, 80
Blank, L.L., 220
Blatt, b., 30
Boex, J.R., 220
Borenstein, B.D., 19, 88, 91, 165, 178
Boulet, J.R., 70

Boulis, A., 31
Brainard, G., 164
Brainard, G.C., 176
Brigham, T.P., 71, 73, 92, 118–120, 148
Brose, J., 42
Brown, A.M., 167
Bu, P., 137
Bucher, J.T., 138
Buffone, A.E.K., 221

C
Callahan, C.A., 4, 6, 14–16, 33, 41, 57, 90, 92,
    98, 139, 140, 149, 196, 221
Caltone, M.P., 213
Carline, J., 69
Carter-Nolan, P.L., 30
Caruso, J.W., 64, 217, 218
Case, S.M., 69
Cass, J., 217
Cass, J.L., 221
Christian, E.D., 33, 35
Cicchetti, A., 197
Clauser, B.E., 56
Cochran, C., 107, 109, 110
Cohen, M., 163
Cohen, M.J.M., 189, 190, 207, 209
Collier, V.U., 96
Conly, S. Jr., 12
Cooter, R., 140
Croiset, G., 230
Crutchley, P., 221

© The Author(s), under exclusive license to Springer Nature Switzerland AG 2022   247
J. S. Gonnella et al., *Fifty Years of Findings from the Jefferson Longitudinal
Study of Medical Education*, https://doi.org/10.1007/978-3-030-85379-2

D
Daitch, Z., 219
Damjanov, I., 141, 159
Darby, E., 21–22
DeCleene-Do, H., 30
DeSantis, J., 167, 174, 186, 187
Diamond, J.J., 22, 105, 106, 127, 175
Dillon, G.F., 56
Doria, C., 154

E
Eichstaedt, J.C., 221
Eidelman, S., 197
Eiger, G., 68
Erdmann, J.B., 4, 6, 16, 32, 36, 50, 51, 57,
        82–85, 89, 90, 92, 94, 96, 98, 99, 103,
        140, 150, 152, 153, 161, 162, 171, 173,
        196, 207, 208, 210, 214, 229

F
Fascelli, M., 219
Fassihi, R., 211
Feeney, K., 158
Fenderson, B.A., 141
Ferretti, S., 108
Fields, S.K., 101, 123, 126, 129, 183,
        188–190, 197, 209, 220
Forouzan, I., 97
Friedman, M., 69
Frisby, A.J., 210

G
Garcia, A., 209
Gartland, J., 33
Geva, H., 197
Glaser, K., 5, 15, 35, 36, 148, 159
Glaser, K.M., 151
Goepp, C.E., 5, 8, 79, 80, 178
Gonnella, J., 230
Gonnella, J.S., 4, 13, 14, 16, 36–40, 45, 50,
        51, 53, 57, 60, 61, 64, 67, 81–86, 89,
        90, 92–96, 98–100, 103, 104, 114, 122,
        139, 140, 142, 149, 150, 152–154, 156,
        158–161, 164, 183, 186, 188, 191–200,
        203–208, 210–214, 216, 218, 225, 226,
        229, 232
Gottheil, E., 148
Gottlieb, J., 60, 101
Gottlieb, J.E., 64, 162
Gottlieb, R.P., 64
Greeson, J.M., 176

Griffiths, M., 189, 190, 209
Grinberg, C., 66

H
Hafferty, F., 168
Hasbrouck, C., 69
Hazelwood, C.E., 22, 105
Heil, D., 30
Herman, M.W., 17, 34, 87, 93, 102, 143–
        145, 201
Herrine, S.K., 164
Hodgson, C.S., 231
Hojat, M., 4–16, 18–19, 22, 24, 25, 30, 32, 33,
        35–45, 50–53, 55, 57, 58, 60, 61, 63, 64,
        79–92, 94–99, 101, 103, 104, 107–110,
        114, 119–123, 127–131, 138–142,
        145–167, 169, 171–174, 176–178,
        182–219, 221, 225, 226, 228–230, 232

I
Ibarra, D., 162, 197, 209
Ibarra, G., 209
Isenberg, G., 163, 167
Isenberg, G.A., 59, 164, 211

J
Jacobs, J., 31
Jafari, N., 16
Johnson, J.J., 109
Jones, R.L., 107, 110
Julian, E., 6
Jung, J., 30

K
Kane, G., 205
Kane, G.C., 183, 206, 218
Kanter, S.L., 107, 109, 110
Kelliher, G.J., 108
Kellow, W.F., 93
Knettler, T.R., 231
Kowitt, B., 154
Kowlessar, D., 178
Kusurkar, R.A., 230

L
Lamberton, C.E., 217
Lane, J.L., 64
LaNoue, M., 202
Liva, C., 197

Lo Sasso, A.A., 217
Lo Scalzo, A., 197
Lopreiato, J., 30
Louis, D.Z., 60, 61, 64, 90, 98, 152, 160, 162,
    203, 204
Lyons, K., 155

M
Macinati, M., 197
Maclaren, C., 69
Magee, M., 156, 158, 183, 195, 196, 198, 199,
    207, 208, 216
Maio, V., 204
Majdan, J., 66
Majdan, J.F., 55, 70, 182
Mancall, E.L., 85
Mangione, S., 156, 183, 185, 195–196, 198,
    199, 205–208, 216, 218
Markham, F.W., 60, 61, 64, 105, 106
Markle, R.A., 16
Mashiach, T., 197
Maxwell, K., 164, 203
Michalec, B., 157, 168, 169
Mochen, E., 108
Modi, A., 219
Morrison, G., 108
Moses, S.L., 65, 104

N
Nasca, T., 205, 214
Nasca, T.J., 6, 33, 57, 64, 68, 90, 92, 96, 152,
    156, 158, 171, 195–199, 205, 207–210,
    214, 216, 218
Nash, D.B., 41
Neimeyer, G.J., 213
Ney, D.B., 187
Nicholson, S., 170
Novielli, K., 40, 171

O
Owens, T., 30

P
Papadakis, M.A., 231
Park, P.K., 40
Pascual, R., 158
Paskin, D.L., 68, 90
Paynter, N.P., 106
Peck, J., 6
Plumb, J.D., 189, 190

Pohl, C.A., 52, 62, 172, 174
Politzer, R.M., 130, 131

R
Rabinowitz, C., 60, 61, 64
Rabinowitz, H.K., 20–22, 63, 105–110, 130,
    131, 175
Raimondo, R., 173
Rattner, S., 131
Rattner, S.L., 36, 52, 57, 61, 64, 70, 96,
    107–111, 123, 130, 152, 161, 189, 208,
    209, 231
Reibel, D.K., 176
Ricciardi, G., 197
Rimoldi, H.J.A., 173
Robeson, M., 70
Robeson, M.R., 19, 39, 52, 62, 68, 92,
    107–111, 117, 119, 159
Rodgers, J.F., 71, 118
Rodgers, J.S., 65
Rosenfeld, L.M., 8
Rosenthal, M.P., 175
Rosenthal, S., 66, 174
Rosenthal, S.R., 221
Rosenzweig, S., 176
Roy, V., 59
Rubin, E., 141
Russo, S., 66

S
Sachs, L., 116
Sammon, M., 217
Schaeffer, A., 30
Schlussel, Y., 174
Schwartz, A., 221
Schwartz, G.F., 67
Seltezer, J.L., 113
Seltzer, J.L., 112, 113
Sierles, F.S., 114
Silber, C.G., 68, 115
Silenzio, V.M.B., 127
Smith, L.K., 221
Spandorfer, J., 160, 163, 185, 211, 215
Sterling, G., 108
Stern, D.T., 231
Swanson, D.B., 69

T
Tangucci, M., 197
Taroni, F., 197
Taylor, J.M., 213

Teherani, A., 231
Torres-Ruiz, A., 197, 209
Trayes, K., 174
Turner, B.J., 53
Turner, T.N., 175
Tykocinski, M.L., 157, 169

U
Ungar, L.H., 221
Urbano, F., 158

V
Van Winkle, L.J., 215
Veloski, J., 4, 55, 94, 113, 214
Veloski, J.A., 56
Veloski, J.J., 5–12, 14, 16, 17, 19, 23–25, 30–32,
    34–37, 39–45, 51, 52, 54, 56–59, 62,
    64–73, 82–93, 95, 96, 99–104, 107–112,
    115–131, 137, 145, 148, 151, 152, 157,
    159, 161, 162, 164, 167–169, 171, 177,
    182, 190, 196, 198, 200, 205, 207, 210,
    212, 213, 220, 226, 229, 231, 232
Vergare, M., 163, 164
Vergare, M.J., 114, 199, 211, 216
Vogel, W.H., 153, 165
Vu, D.M., 138

W
Waechter, D., 69
Ward, J., 215
Williams, B., 215
Williams, T., 116
Wilson, J., 66
Winward, M., 56
Wolfson, P.J., 117
Worzala, K., 70

X
Xu, G., 14, 36–39, 41–45, 54, 71–73,
    103, 107–110, 118–131, 140,
    148, 162

Y
Yaden, D.B., 221
Yaden, M.B., 174
Yaden, M.E., 221
Yeo, C.J., 59

Z
Zeleznik, C., 7, 9–14, 24, 25, 86, 93, 165,
    177, 178
Zuckerman, M., 166, 216

Subject Index

A

Academic performances, 45, 140, 153, 159, 172, 196
Academic performances of geriatricians, 126
Academic preparation
  baccalaureate preparation, 24
  career plan, 13
  combined BS-MD degree program, 16
  demographics, 22
  economic factor, 22
  Empathy Score in Admission Decisions, 18
  letters of recommendation, 25
  medical school performances, 13
  Penn State-Jefferson Accelerated Program, 14
  performance, 17
  personal characteristics, 17
  postbaccalaureate preparation, 19
  postgraduate clinical performance, 23
  prematriculation enrichment program, 15
  premedical training, 17
  PSAP, 21
  retention, 22
  undergraduate majors, 13
  underserved areas, 20
Accreditation Council for Graduate Medical Education (ACGME)
  competencies, 68
Adulthood, 146
Affirmative action, 94
African-American, 30, 33, 41
Age, 32, 36, 41
Allied health students, 155
AMA Physicians' Professional Data (AMA-PPD), 115
AMEE Guide 79, 150
American Medical Association, 117
Anesthesiology, 31, 112, 113
Argentina, 173
Asian-American, 41, 42, 45
Asian/Pacific Islander, 30, 43
Assessment measures
  medical school, residency training and practice, 84
Association for the Study of Medical Education (ASME), 18

B

Baccalaureate preparation, 24
Beck Depression Inventory, 151
Biotechnology, 142, 195
Board certification, 39, 44, 85, 89, 94, 115, 126
Burnout, 163

C

Career choice, 101, 103, 110, 116, 125, 127, 140, 148
Career data, 226
Career plan, 13
Career satisfaction, 154
Change of interest, 40
Childhood, 146
chi-square tests, 45
Class ranking, 79, 80, 99
Clerkship experiences on students' satisfaction, 72
Clinical competence, 50, 53, 57, 67, 68, 149, 196

Clinical judgment, 93
Clinical performance, 63
Clinical skills (CS), 56, 66
Clinician empathy, 186
Cognitive factors, 88
Collaborative education, 209
Combined BS-MD degree program, 16
Communication skills, 217
Components of competence, 88, 90, 91
Comprehensive examination, 58
Conceptualization, 160
Conceptualization and measurement, 92
Confirmatory factor analysis (CFA), 202
Content and context of performance, 225
Core clerkships, 57
Correlational analyses, 90
COVID-19, 187
Criterion-related validity, 92
Critics, 200
Cronbach's coefficient, 191
Curriculum modification, 65

D

Data gathering and processing skills, 91, 93
Delayed graduation, 8, 13, 50
Demographics, 22
Disability Attitudes in Health Care (DAHC)
        scale, 137
Disciplinary action, 231
Dismissal rates, 51
Distress, 174
Documentation of clinical experiences,
        60, 61, 64
Dying patients, 187

E

Early career specialization, 99
Early specialization, 100
Economic diversity, 140
Economic factor, 22
Educational debt, 140
Electronic medical records (EMRs), 217
Emergency medicine (EM), 31, 99, 117, 121,
        124, 125, 128
Emotional Instability, 151
Empathic and sympathetic orientations, 160
Empathic behavior, 156
Empathic engagement, 204, 228
Empathy, 55, 68, 157, 163, 172, 228
    academic performance, 196
    clinical competence, 196
    cognitive attribute, 200
    cognitive nature, 204

critics, 200
definition, 184, 204
dying patients, 187
empirical research, 208
enhancing and sustaining, 185
gender, 196
health professionals, 183
internal medicine training, 218
IRI, 194
Jefferson Scale of Physician Empathy, 198
JSPE *vs.* IRI, 206
linguistic analysis, 221
medical education, 193, 205
medical school, 184
medical students, 208
NODA program, 187
NP/MD comparison, 188
patient care, 193, 205, 207
patient outcomes, 183
patient perceptions, clinician's
        empathy, 186
patient-physician relationships, 196
perceptions of, 216
personality, 216
physician, 195, 204
specialty interest, 203, 216
SPs, 182
student-run free clinics and changes, 219
Empathy Score in Admission Decisions, 18
Empathy scores, 156
Enhancement of Empathy, 185
Entire-group prediction model, 32
Erosion of empathy, 164, 184, 200
Ethnicity, 30
Exploratory factor analysis (EFA), 202
Extraversion, 151

F

Faculty members, 101
Faculty ratings, 57, 66
Failure rate, 66
Family income, 140
Family medicine career, 97, 99, 100, 102, 105,
        110, 116, 121, 126, 128
Family medicine clerkship, 61
Family physicians, 105, 118, 126
Family practice, 31
Financial aid, 127
F-tests, 45

G

Gender, 30–33, 35–40, 196
Gender comparisons, 35, 36, 38, 39, 96, 123

Gender segregation, 31
General surgery residency programs, 117
Generalist, 107
Generalist career, 101, 109, 110, 123, 127
Generalist Physician Initiative (GPI), 108
Generalist physicians, 107, 127
Geriatricians, 126
Grade-point averages (GPAs), 15, 121
Grading systems, 50
Graduate medical education (GME), 107
Grit, 167

H
Healthcare costs, 37
Healthcare environment, 162
Healthcare system, 93, 96, 143, 144, 152,
    161, 162
Health services research, 98
History-taking skills, 217
Honors Program in Pathology, 141

I
Imposter phenomenon (IP), 174
Income expectations, 34, 36, 40, 175, 177
Inner city and rural areas, 104–106, 127, 130, 131
Insurance and governmental regulations, 225
Interdisciplinary education, 189, 211
Internal medicine, 31, 81
Interpersonal dimension, 118
Interpersonal Reactivity Index (IRI), 160,
    194, 206
Interpersonal relationships of physicians, 145
Interpersonal skills, 79, 88, 89, 91, 92, 119
Interprofessional collaboration and teamwork,
    197, 209, 211, 215

J
Jefferson empathy research, 228
Jefferson Health Care System, 205
Jefferson Longitudinal Study (JLS),
    226–229, 232
Jefferson Longitudinal Study of Medical
    Education (JLSME), 31, 230, 232
Jefferson Medical College (JMC), 22, 116
Jefferson scale of attitudes toward
    interprofessional collaboration
    (JEFFSATIC), 215
Jefferson Scale of Empathy (JSE), 18, 160,
    184, 185, 194, 200, 203, 217, 228
    CFA, 202
    EFA, 202
    gender difference, 203

Jefferson Scale of Empathy-Medical Student
    version (JSE-S), 192
Jefferson Scale of Patient Perceptions of
    Physician Empathy (JSPPPE), 30,
    55, 182, 186, 200
Jefferson Scale of Physician Empathy (JSPE),
    182, 183, 188, 195, 196, 198, 199,
    206–208, 216, 218
Jefferson Scale of Physician Lifelong Learning
    (JeffSPLL), 212–214

K
Knowledge acquisition examination, 51, 53,
    58, 63, 67, 68
Knowledge and Clinical Capabilities, 90
Knowledge, data gathering, and processing
    skills, 92

L
Legal-economic dimension, 118
Letters of recommendation, 25
Liaison Committee on Medical Education
    (LCME), 232
Lifelong learning, 210
Linguistic analysis, 221
Low ratings, 87

M
Managed care, 161
Maternal care, 146
Measurement, 160
Measures of clinical skills, 85, 103
Medical College Admission Test
    (MCAT), 5, 16, 17, 41, 43, 45,
    141, 159
    medical school, residency and licensing
        examinations, 4
    NBE, 5
    overall validity, 9
    science subtest scores and
        performance, 12
    scores, 7
    undergraduate institutions, 11
    writing sample section, 6
Medical education, 205, 230, 231
    ultimate goal, 225
Medical education and patient care, 79,
    86, 88–90
Medical education curriculum, 229
Medical education outcomes, 225, 229
Medical licensing examinations, 50, 51, 226
Medical school applicants, 32

Medical school evaluations
　clinical
　　ACGME competencies, 68
　　activities and learning experiences, 65
　　attending physicians and residents, 71
　　clerkship experiences on students'
　　　satisfaction, 72
　　clinical performance, 63
　　comprehensive examination, 58
　　core clerkships, 57
　　CS, 56, 66
　　curriculum modification, 65
　　documentation of clinical
　　　experiences, 64
　　empathy, 55
　　faculty ratings, 57
　　failure rate, 66
　　family medicine clerkship, 61
　　gender differences, 60
　　knowledge acquisition
　　　examination, 58, 67
　　modified essay examination, 63
　　objective examinations, 67
　　overall satisfaction, 54
　　performance assessments, 58, 62, 67
　　residency supervisor ratings, 57
　　retention, 58
　　role of residents, 54
　　self-assessments, 59
　　SPs, 55, 59
　　standardized patient, 70
　　students' active involvement, 73
　preclinical
　　grading systems, 50
　　levels of knowledge, 51
　　NBME examinations, 53
　　performance administration, 52
　　physician competence, 51
　　predictive validity, 50
　　residency supervisor ratings, 53
　　test administration, 52
　　USMLE (see United States Medical
　　　Licensing Examination (USMLE))
Medical school performances, 13
Medical schools, 225, 226, 231
Medicine, 225
Men and women physicians, 123
Middle States Commission on Higher
　　Education, 232
Mindfulness-based stress reduction
　　(MBSR), 176
Mirror neuron system (MNS), 204
Mistaken identity, 82
Modified essay examination, 63

Multi-institutional study, 30
Multiple regression, 90

N
Narratives, 231
National and international medical education
　　researchers, 84
National Board, 33
National Board Examination (NBE), 5, 9,
　　88, 95, 100
National Board of Medical Examinations
　　(NBME), 7, 9, 11, 12, 19, 24, 25,
　　32, 43, 45, 53, 63, 81, 89, 99, 116,
　　121, 124, 126, 128
National Board scores, 117
Neurons, 204
Noise, 82
Noncognitive areas, 87
Noncognitive factors, 88
Noncognitive measures, 87
Non-primary care, 103, 119
Non-PSAP students, 20

O
Objective examinations, 67
Objective Structured Clinical Examination
　　(OSCE), 66, 182
Obstetrics and gynecology, 31, 81, 97, 115
Ohio State University College of Medicine
　　(OSU), 116
Ophthalmology, 31
Optimism, 163
Orthopedic surgeons, 118
Overall satisfaction, 54, 73

P
Pass/fail (P/F) grades, 50, 69
Pathology, 31
Patient care, 205
Patient encounters, 60, 61, 64
Patient perceptions, 186
Pediatricians, 118
Pediatrics, 31, 81
Peer nomination, 157, 168, 172
Penn State-Jefferson Accelerated
　　Program, 14
Pennsylvania model, 108
People-oriented specialties, 148
Performance administration, 52
Performance and career expectations of
　　women, 34

Performance assessment, 50–52, 56–59, 62, 66, 69, 82
Personality, 153, 172
Personality and specialty interest, 166
Personality assessment, 150
Personality factors, 138
Personality profiles, 158
Pertinent personal qualities, 225
PGY-1 programs, 117
Pharmacist-physician collaborative relationships, 191
Physical well-being, 153
Physician competence, 5, 51
Physician empathy
  biotechnology, 195
  components, 199
  definition, 199
  gender and specialty relationship, 199
  medical school admission essays, 221
  patient care, 195
Physician empathy measurement, 199
Physician income, 170
Physician roles and responsibilities, 142
Physician Shortage Area Program (PSAP), 20, 21, 105, 106
Physician unionization, 96
Physicians' lifelong learning
  assessment, 214
  conceptualization, 213
  full-time clinicians and academic clinicians, 213
  measurement, 212, 213
  psychometric properties, 210
Positive influencers, 157, 169
Postgraduate and career
  clinical competence
    affirmative action, 94
    assessment measures, 84
    board certification, 85
    class ranking, 79, 80
    cognitive factors, 88
    components of competence, 90, 91
    conceptualization and measurement, 92
    learning, 83
    longitudinal data, 83
    medical education and patient care, 86
    medical school and postgraduate competence, 81
    National Board Examination, 95
    noncognitive areas, 87
    noncognitive factors, 88
    performance assessment, 82
    performance in medical school and first postgraduate year, 93

preferential admission, 94
psychometric evaluation, 79, 80
reexamination, 89
resident's performance, 85
specialization and professional activities
  academic performances of geriatricians, 126
  anesthesiology, 113
  assessment of physicians, 111
  board certification, 115
  career choice, 110, 116, 127
  changing specialties, 112
  early career specialization, 99
  early specialization, 100
  EM, 121, 124, 125
  family medicine career, 102, 121, 128
  family physicians, 105, 118
  financial aid, 127
  general surgery residency programs, 117
  generalist career, 109, 110
  generalist physicians, 107, 127
  GPI, 108
  health services research, 98
  healthcare system, 122
  inner city and rural areas, 105, 131
  migration of physicians, 113
  NBME Part II examination, 116
  non-primary care, 103, 119
  obstetrics-gynecology, 97
  orthopedic surgeons, 118
  pediatricians, 118
  perceptions of professional problems, 104
  personal characteristics, 127
  physician unionization, 96
  practice patterns between men and women graduates, 104
  primary care, 101–103, 119, 120, 123, 129, 130
  psychiatrists' academic performance, 114
  rural primary care practice and retention, 106
  stability and change, 97
  student characteristics, 102
  trends, 102
  underserved areas, 105
Postgraduate clinical performance, 23
Postgraduate competence, 79–81, 89, 90
Potential leaders, 157
Practice patterns between men and women graduates, 104
Predictive validity, 4, 7, 11, 50

Preferential admission, 94
Preferential selection, 20
Prematriculation enrichment program, 15
Premedical training, 17
Primary care, 101–103, 105, 106, 110, 111,
       119, 120, 123, 125–131
Primary care career choice, 42
Primary care training/retraining, 111
Professional accomplishments, 154
Professional activities, 104
Professional attitudes, 145
Professional careers, 33
Professionalism, 90, 231
    communication skills, 217
    cross-cultural comparisons, 209
    empathy (*see* Empathy)
    EMR-specific communication, 217
    history-taking skills, 217
    interprofessional collaboration, 215
    lifelong learning, 210, 212–214
    measurement, physicians' lifelong
        learning, 212
    measures, 220
    medical responsibility, 189
    physician authority, 189
    physician-nurse alliances, 189
    physician-nurse collaboration, 190, 191,
        197, 209
    physician-pharmacist collaboration, 211
    physicians' attitudes toward nurse
        perceptions, 201
    proxy norm data, 192
    students' empathy, 182
    tentative cutoff scores, 192
Profile of Mood States (POMS), 176
Prototype of assessment, 229
Psychiatrists' academic performance, 114
Psychiatry, 31
Psychological attributes
    academic performance, 140
    biotechnology and ethics, 142
    burnout, 163
    career choice, 140, 148
    career satisfaction, 154
    characteristics, 155, 159
    clinical competence, 149
    distress, 174
    early relationships with parents and adults'
        psychosocial attributes, 147
    economic aspects, 144
    economic diversity, 140
    educational debt, 140
    empathic and sympathetic orientations, 160
    empathic behavior, 156
    empathy, 163
    empathy scores, 156
    erosion of empathy, 164
    family income, 140
    grit, 167
    healthcare system, 152, 161
    Honors Program in Pathology, 141
    income expectations, 175, 177
    interpersonal relationships of
        physicians, 145
    intra- and intercultural similarities and
        differences on personality
        profiles, 173
    IP, 174
    managed care, 161
    maternal care, 146
    MBSR, 176
    opinions concerning of healthcare
        system, 143
    optimism, 163
    PAS, 171
    peer nomination, 168, 172
    perceptions of medical school seniors, 162
    personality and specialty interest, 166
    personality assessment, 150
    personality factors, 138
    personality profiles, 158
    physician clinical competence
        ratings, 151
    physician income, 170
    positive influencers, 157, 169
    potential leaders, 157
    professional accomplishments, 154
    professional attitudes, 145
    psychostimulant drugs, 138
    PWDs, 137
    role model, 158
    social network approach, 168
    stressful life events, 147, 153, 165
    student debt, 140
    students' certainty, 178
    students' personality, 149
    volunteer bias, 139
Psychometric evaluation, 79, 80
Psychometrics, 155, 160
Psychosocial measures, 88
Psychosocial profiles, 35
Psychostimulant drugs, 138

Q
Quantitative skills, 5

R
Radiology, 31
Ratings of clerkships, 65
Reexamination, 89
Research activities, 33
Residency supervisor ratings, 51, 53, 57
Resident's performance, 85
Retention, 22, 51, 58
Role model, 158
Rosenberg Self-Esteem Scale, 151
Rural primary care practice and
        retention, 106

S
Salary inequities, 37
Satisfaction with medical school, 33
Scholastic Aptitude Test (SAT)
    long-range predictive and differential
        validities, 10
Science skills, 5
Selection of applicants, 18, 20
Self-assessments, 59
Signal, 82
Simulated patients (SPs), 55, 59, 182
Social accountability, 225
Social network approach, 168
Social role theory, 197
Socioeconomic dimensions, 91
Specialty interest, 103, 172
Standardized patient (SP), 30, 70, 217
Standardized tests
    delayed graduation, 8
    long-range predictive and differential
        validities, 10
    MCAT (*see* Medical College Admission
        Test (MCAT))
    overall validity, 9
    predictive validity, 7
    quantitative skills, 5
    science skills, 5
    Undergraduate institutions, 11
    verbal skills, 5
    writing sample section, 6

Stressful life events, 147, 153, 165, 173
Student characteristics, 102
Student debt, 140
Student-run free clinic, 219
Students' certainty, 178
Students' personality, 149
Surgery, 31
Sustaining empathy, 185
Sympathy, 193, 204

T
Targeted educational programs, 228
Taylor Manifest Anxiety Scale, 151
Technology-oriented specialties, 148
Total mood disturbance (TMD), 176
Trends, 102
t-test, 90
Types of unprofessional behavior, 231

U
UCLA Loneliness, 151
Undergraduate grade point average, 8,
        11, 19, 24
Undergraduate institutions, 11, 12, 25
Undergraduate majors, 13, 17, 24
Underrepresented minority (URM), 40, 42, 44
Underserved areas, 20, 21, 104, 105, 130
United States Medical Licensing Examination
        (USMLE), 52, 56, 62, 66, 69, 141
Unprofessional behavior, 231
US healthcare system, 122

V
Verbal skills, 5
Volunteer bias, 139
Volunteerism, 219

W
White physicians, 33
Writing Sample section, 6